WHAT A COMEBACK!

THE LAWS THAT CHANGE THE WAY WE THINK

DR.CHIRAG JAIN

Book Title: What a Comeback!
Book Author: Dr.Chirag.B.Jain

Published by Dr. Chirag B Jain
417 Chandralok B Bldg. manav mandir road
Walkeshwar
Published in Mumbai, India

Printed and bound by Dr. Chirag Jain
417 Chandralok B Bldg manav mandir road
Walkeshwar
Mumbai, India

This edition published August 2018

ISBN 9789353119041
Copyright © Dr.Chirag B Jain 2018

For
Dr.V.P.Shanmughasundaram M.S

You would love to read it, Sir.

Contents

The degree of attention is directly proportional to the mental force of a thought.

Minds like other planets and organism tends to function in automations. It is the level of awareness that enables us to break these automations and make conscious and path breaking decisions. The more the mind functions in automations the more are the misery and unhappiness it experiences.

The more the mind functions in automation the more are the

misery and unhappiness it experiences **.**

In our pursuit to mix automations with awareness we have developed from part of the creation to so called rulers of creation…..in the journey we have migrated from being a part of stillness of nature to the slayers of our own peace and tranquillity.

The more we are aware of these automations in the mind, the lesser fuel we give to these Chapter pathways to become rigid and fixed. The more fixed and rigid our thinking, the lesser we are in control of our behaviours and reactions.

Awareness is a habit difficult to cultivate because of mans greed for social interactions.

Note to the Readers

My intention of writing the book is to reach
people of varied streams who may not like to read
the science section. Hence, the science part has
been highlighted in the form of italic font.
Happy Reading!

Acknowledgment

It's been a roller coaster ride for me to reach to a point where I have written this book and formulated the laws. There have been many people which have inspired me, stood by me. At the outset, I would like to acknowledge all of them for inspiring me to write this book.

I would like to thank my parents who have stood by me, every moment, when life was not so simple and straight. I am grateful to them for being the backbone for me, so I could come to a stage where I can question the status quo.I am indebted to my loving wife, Darshana for standing with me and always inspiring me to write this book. She has stood by my side and has always pushed me every second, when I wanted to give up. Your criticisms are the inspirations which helped me complete my first book.

My children Jiya and Dveep whose freshness of thoughts always make me go beyond my expectations.

I would like to thank Manish Sisodia the deputy chief minister of New Delhi, India for inspiring me to come with my own theory of neuroplasticity and write a book on it. It isn't every day you thank a politician for inspiring you. His simplicity and straightforwardness prompted me to think about the concept of neuroplasticity and work towards analysing the thought process of the human mind.

Above all, I would like to thank my patients and students, who have always been kind enough to support me. I am indebted to each one of them for their patience in dealing with me.

I would like to thank Dave Potter who introduced
me to the world of mindfulness. If it weren't for
his program on mindfulness, I would have never
tried to explore new avenues.
I would like to thank all the authors and
neuroplasticians who had laid the foundation
stone in my quest for understanding the process of
neuroplasticity. Highly grateful to Daniel
Goldman, Norman Doidge, Jeffrey.M.Schwartz
and David Rock whose books have inspired me to
understand the subject

In the end, I would like to conclude that the
purpose for writing the book will be
accomplished if it can make a difference in the
life of a single individual and redefine the fixed
and rigid neural pathways which are creating a
hindrance in their personal or work relationship.

Preface

It was a cold winter day, somewhere in the month of December in Mumbai, India in the year 2014. I was returning from my clinic after having a hectic day of consultation. Although I was tired, I had to attend a family get-to-gather at a restaurant which had recently opened in town. This was one of the rare occasions when I was able to reach on time as I had strict instructions from my family. Being a Saturday night, the restaurant was jam-packed. I located my family's table. Everyone was surprised at me being on time. It was a long time since I had met them.

I was getting disturbed by a lady's voice. Turning my attention to the table, I overheard a very interesting conversation between a mother and a sixteen-year-old teenage girl. The mother was recollecting the daughter's mistakes and shortcomings, and how they will be affecting her future. She had a never-ending, long list and the teenager was simply staring at her in disbelief and disgust. She tried to interrupt but it seemed that the mother was well-prepared and her tirade of complaints were simply not stopping. When the mother ran out of words, the teenager shot back with a calm tone "Mom if there are so many issues, could you also give me the solution for them. Before you interrupt me, you can also tell me what was the root cause of these issues and what did you do about it for the last sixteen years? Also, would you also want me to point out the problems which I have inherited from you, out of the long list you have told me?" Her mother was shocked at her daughter's candid and frank reply

to her onslaught. More than anger she realised
what she said was making sense. She looked at
her daughter timidly as a small girl who is caught
red-handed by someone doing mischief. She told
her that she had realised that her daughter had
grown up. Any mother wouldn't want her
daughter to go through the same problems.
This conversation was like any other conversation
between teenage kids and their parents. However,
this made me realise that there was a lot more
meaning in what the kid was trying to tell her
parent. As a parent of two children, I do
understand that all parents try to teach kids, skills
and behaviours, so they can be better human
beings and face the harsh realities of life boldly
.Is parenting only responsible for the teen's
behaviour? Does the society have a role?
On researching further I realised the complexity
of a teenagers mind. The effect on their mind
because of the bombardment of information, as
they enters adult life. I had always been well
versed with the anatomy of the brain, but as I
dived deeper into the newer research done by
neuroscientist worldwide, a whole new world of
the mind and its functioning opened up in front of
me. Reading through not only a neuroscientist
point of view, also the perspective of
neurophysics and psychology made me see the
broader picture. How the new neurons are created
and the properties which govern the formation of
these new pathways?
I started studying behaviours of my students and
tried to analyse the process of comeback. I
realised that there are many issues which were

half explained or left out and felt there was a void in individual understanding about the process of comeback. So I formulated the findings into ten different laws to make the process of comeback more explainable. There are old habits and behaviours which are interfering in our life and most individuals. Some have defined this as fixed thinking. How this fixed thinking affects our decision- making? Why our mind gets so tempted to get into a mode of fixed thinking? What is the role of Mindfulness in modulating thought processes?

 It has always been possible to deal with these complex circuits of a human mind and overcome a fixed mind set for some individuals. However there are many who struggle as they get entangled into difficult situations.
Based on these laws I have devised a strategy using 4'Rs mainly **Realization, Raising an anchor, Rewiring and Redefining**. Mindfulness and its role in Neuroplasticity also came as a revelation to me as I saw remarkable changes in people who enrolled with me in the program. I realised that it was possible for everyone to overcome their behavioural issues caused by these automated pathways. The 4R strategy is more attuned to the laws which are formulated and form the essence of the interventions.
The next hindrance which was pointed out to me by most of the people was that although the laws are one or two sentences long, they were difficult to understand and relate to their life. Hence, the laws have been explained in the form of individual stories of triumph of day to day life.

All the stories are interconnected and are happening in the same time period. The book narrates the stories about Sam and his old mates who goes through a torrid time integrity life and how they comeback from those situations. It takes the reader on a journey inside each and every character's mind and how they get entangled in a situation.

In the end, I would like to conclude, that the purpose of writing the book will be accomplished if it can make a difference in the life of a single individual and redefine the fixed and rigid neural pathway, paving way for a comeback.

Laws of Neuroplasticity ©
1. The degree of attention is directly proportional to the mental force of a thought.
2. Minds like other planets and organism tend to function in automation. It is the level of awareness that enables us to break this automation and make conscious and path-breaking decisions.
3. The more the mind functions in automation the more are the misery and unhappiness it experiences.
4. The default state of the mind is awareness i.e. is happiness….it's the inclination and dependence of the mind to save the information and relate it to the emotions generated gives rise to turbulence and noise in a human mind. The more we believe in what we feel rather than what it is, the more unhappiness we generate.
5. Being positive is directly related to the extent of being aware of the moment.

6. Competitive neuroplasticity is a phenomenon taking place every moment of our life and is highly underrated by our experiences.

7. The more the mind believes in the images it forms and the related past emotions the more the sufferings. The lesser it believes in the images it forms the more the scope for awareness and resolving difficult situations.

8. In our pursuit to mix automation with awareness, we have developed from part of the creation to so-called rulers of creation….in the journey we have migrated from being a part of stillness of nature to the slayers of our own peace and tranquillity.

9. The more we are aware of this automation in the mind, the lesser fuel we give to these brain pathways to become rigid and fixed. The more fixed and rigid our thinking, the lesser we are in control of our behaviours and reactions.

10. Awareness is a habit difficult to cultivate because of man's greed for social interactions.

What's the science, Dude?

As the name suggests, most of the readers probably think that this is one of the science books and will have a lot of theories and formulas. Well, there is a bit of surprise in it. I have attempted to explain these laws using real-life stories. Although the primary goal of the book is to impart scientific knowledge, it is simplified to explain various processes involving the working of the human brain and its related neurological processes. An initial understanding of the human brain will make it easier for us to understand Sam and his friend's journey.
This chapter is the only chapter solely dedicated to explain the human brain and understanding the neuronal processes.
Let me start with the revolution which came in the field of neuroscience last decade. We have been taught from a very young age that when we are born, we have the maximum number of cells and as we grow older, cells start decreasing or dying. Also, we believe that the brain is hard-wired and acts and functions in a predetermined way, with areas dedicated to individual functions. All these theories have been recently challenged and proven wrong.
Another theory in the 90s was that genetics decide on what we think, and we feel. Throughout 1980 and 1990 there were many press reports of how twins separated by birth exhibited the similar trait. It was a well-accepted fact that genetics hardwired our mind.
Interestingly since the last decade with advances

in imaging, it was revealed that the brain is plastic in nature. Plastic as in 'it is bendable' and can be modified with our experiences. So what does that mean? The brain keeps changing every moment depending on our experiences. Also, genes layout the potentials and vulnerabilities a person may face but it cannot decide your emotions, your thoughts and ultimately your behaviour. Another surprise is that you can modulate your genes to an extent, with your behaviour.

These new discoveries along with other make it possible for us to change our behaviour and habits, which was the main inspiration for me to write this book. We can maximise our potentials and minimise our vulnerabilities by making use of these findings. I will be taking you through the journey of first understanding the brain functioning and then the laws governing our mind. How we can apply these laws to our lives, so we can improve our decision making in complex situations. Being in a calm state simply means feeling less tense, less anxious and less noise in the brain.

There are parts of your brain which are responsible for these agitated states while there are others responsible for taming them. The right balance is required to create conditions in the mind for exploring our potentials and being in control of the situations in our life. The understanding of the effects on our memory and insight is essential as we start realising that things do not always happen by chance but there are solid reasons within and outside our body which determine the outcome. My focus in the book is to less presume or assume the outcomes and reasons. I have attempted to try and find out more logical and scientific reasons behind the thought processes and emotions in our body.

Being to Behaviour
We were all born with a brain which was similar structurally and functionally, except the genetic influence on it. As our experiences crept in, our behavioural patterns got defined. Slowly from just being a brain to creating a behavioural pattern, there were many structural changes in the brain and its network. To understand these changes let us know the basic structure of the brain.
The brain weighs just three pounds, yet it's one of the most advanced complicated machines existing in the world today. It has a hundred billion nerve cells called neurons, and many more support cells that are equivalent to the number of stars in our galaxy, that too in a single human brain.
Let's start with the basic structure of the brain. The neurons are clustered in parts of the brain known as modules: the cortex (the outer layers have two hemispheres right and left) the four lobes (frontal, parietal, occipital and temporal) and the subcortical areas (below the cortex).

Right and Left Hemispheres
Lots of hype and jokes have been made on the social media about the functioning of the right and left hemisphere, especially in the context of the male and female brain. Right brain dominant

*people are said to be more creative and spiritual
than the left brain and this hype 'born in 1970'
still exists. However, the truth is that both
hemispheres have to work in tandem for any
activity we do. The brain contains a band of fibres
called as corpus callosum which binds the two
hemispheres together. It serves to connect the
faraway neurons and in layman's words, creates
more depth and understanding. How we
comprehend and understand a situation or a
given text is directly related to the density of these
fibres.*

*The corpus callosum is denser in females than
males. So what does that mean? Hemispheres in
female work more evenly together and in simpler
terms, they have better collaboration. The female
brain is more symmetrical. However, in the male
brain, the right frontal lobe is larger than the left
frontal lobe and the left occipital lobe larger than
the right occipital lobe.*

*Right hemisphere for both sexes processes visual
and spatial information, which helps them to
grasp the "bigger picture". The right hemisphere
gives more weight to the context or the gist of the
situation. Whereas the left is more tuned at fine
details, categories and linearly arranged
information like language. The right fellow is
more activated when we learn something new.
Once the know-how and knowledge are learned,
then the left hemisphere comes more into action
for repeating the process-again and again.
Hence, language is processed by the left
hemisphere.*

The right hemisphere makes better connections

with the subcortical regions and hence is more emotional by nature. To make it simpler, this is responsible for us to understand the emotional part of the conversation. Since women have a better cross-hemispheric connection, they are more intuitive and word spoken by them carry a lot of meaning compared to the male counterpart. Probably this is the reason why women are said to be more emotional.

The four lobes of the brain have specific talents. The speed with which they operate in every single moment is simply phenomenal and here is where we realise, why the brain is called the supercomputer. For example, you remember a meeting an old friend a few days back in a hotel… you appreciate the beautiful ambiance of the hotel when you went with him, particularly the sofa. You recollect the shape of the sofa by activating the parietal lobe. When you remember the words of your friend "what you did in good old school times" you process the temporal lobe. When you recollect looking back and seeing a beautiful lady seated behind your sofa, you use the occipital lobe.

However, women have a greater density of neurons in the temporal lobe that specialises in language. What does that mean? Well, the verbal advantage in female begins to appear from the age of two years. Majority of little girls develop the ability to talk six months earlier than little boys do..Verbal strategies are developed in women which activate the left hippocampus (part of the brain related to memory) more than men do. Men, however, have greater visual and spatial skills because they show greater activity in the right hippocampus than women do. It simply means women can recollect the events and describe better, when in a conversation than males who know the content and can visualise the event but find it relatively difficult to describe it.

The frontal lobe also known as the Neo brain makes up 20% of the brain size. In comparison, the cat's frontal lobe, it is only 3% of its brain size. The frontal lobe is the last part of the brain to mature and it sometimes takes three decade for it to fully mature.

The most important part of the frontal lobe is the prefrontal cortex (PFC). This the fellow who gives us our most complex behavioural, cognitive and emotional functions.

The PFC is the one responsible for you to act on your moral need since it lets you put aside your own needs and reflect on what others need. The PFC is involved in the capacity of an individual to be empathetic. People with damaged PFC have antisocial and impulsive behaviour. Lack of purpose is another effect of a damaged or underdeveloped PFC.

Let us go, a little deeper in the understanding of the PFC. The two main principal parts of PFC are dorsolateral prefrontal cortex (DLPFC) and orbitofrontal prefrontal cortex (OFC). The DLPFC is placed on top and side of the brain, as suggested by the name and the OFC is behind occipital and frontal lobe. Most of the anatomical structures are named in relation to the axis which is a central line or in connection with the neighbouring organ, somewhat, like we give

direction using a map.
The DLPFC is responsible for higher-order thinking, attention and short-term or working memory. Working memory is more like the data on the computer which is not saved. You can usually hold to something for twenty to thirty seconds. DLPC is the last part of the brain to develop and the first one to falter in later years of life. This is the fellow responsible when you enter a room purposefully and forget what you intend to do. It is also involved in problem-solving hence has rich connections to the hippocampus which helps you to remember things for later life.
The OFC, in contrast, is more involved with the part of the brain responsible for emotions such as the ones generated by the amygdala (primitive brain responsible for firing emotions). The OFC develops earlier in life and is loosely related to what is called the social brain. To explain it more simply let me talk about Phineas Gage. Phineas Gage had an accident at work where a steel rod pierced Gage's brain and damaged the OFC but left everything intact. Gage retained his cognitive abilities but lost his abilities to control impulses. He was previously a widely respected supervisor who overnight after the incident became an irrational and impulsive person. He was rude, erratic and hard to get along with. He was eventually reduced to working in a circus freak show and died pennilessly. His skull is on display in Harvard Medical School.
The OFC thrives on close relationships. If the relationships are more trustworthy and supportive the OFC becomes more capable of

regulating emotions. However, unlike DLPFC the OFC does not falter with age. Old folks remember faces, as well as the younger ones do. The right PFC develops foresight and gets a gist of what's happening in the given situation. It helps you to make plans stay on course towards your overall goals and understand metaphors. If someone says "Mother Teresa is an angel", it is the right PFC that enables you to understand that this person really is talking about her kindness and compassion. Your left PFC helps you to focus on the details of individual events like how many runs were scored in a cricket match and their individual performances.

Neurochemicals

One thing is clear, that within these hemispheres, lobes and modules there are a hundred billion neurons waiting to be used. Each neuron is highly social and capable of maintaining thousands of connections, like the aunt next door who drops into every house in the building to have a small chit-chat. These are the connections we need, when we learn new things like playing football or learning a language. So let's try to understand the next complex thing in the brain after understanding the structural framework. These neurons connect to each other by electrical impulses and communicate with each other by chemical messengers called neurochemicals across gaps called synapses.

Much like a connector is used when the pin does not fit inside the socket. The only differentiating thing is that there are different sockets for every connection and the current flowing thru them can be regulated. This is how neuron fire and make others fire.

More than sixty types of neurotransmitters exist inside the brain. Some make you excited while other calm you down. There are different size and shapes of synapses, and they change as you learn something.

Two neurotransmitters accounting for 80% of the signals are glutamate which is excitatory and gamma-amino butyric acid (GABA) which is inhibitory and quiets us down. Glutamate is the workforce in our brain. Glutamate functions by initially priming the connection when an electrical current passes and as the connections are repeated again and again, the wiring becomes stronger and stronger. However, GABA acts by calming you down when you need to drugs like Valium and Ativan to act on these transmitters. The other three neurotransmitters of importance are dopamine, serotonin, and norepinephrine and are called as neuromodulators. Neuromodulators alter the sensitivity of the receptors (the place where these neurotransmitters get attached on the synapse) they make the neurons more efficient and instruct the neurons to make more neurotransmitters. These can also help to lower the noise in the brain by overriding the signals that are coming in the synapse. These three can actually act directly like glutamate or GABA or fine tune the flow across the synapses.

Serotonin plays a role in emotional tone and has a varied response in different emotional situations. Low level is correlated with anxiety, depression and OCD (Obsessive Compulsive

Disorder). It is like a traffic cop, which helps us to regulate the brain activity. But over secretions by drugs like Prozac actually make you numb, and you seem to dislike an activity, which previously would make a difference.

Norepinephrine activates attention. It amplifies the signals that influence perception, arousal, and motivation.

Dopamine is associated with sharpening and focusing attention. It is also known as the reward hormone and helps in learning. Pleasure is one of the key emotion activated by dopamine released by an area called nucleus accumbens referred as pleasure centre. Repeated activation of this area is associated with gambling, drug abuse, and other addictive behaviour.

A sense of self-triumph which in today's world, we call it as ego and enforcing our views on others is another example of attempt of human brain to relive the experience by stimulating the dopamine release. Of course, the argument which follows that it can also be activated due to our amygdala (danger detecting brain) getting activated.

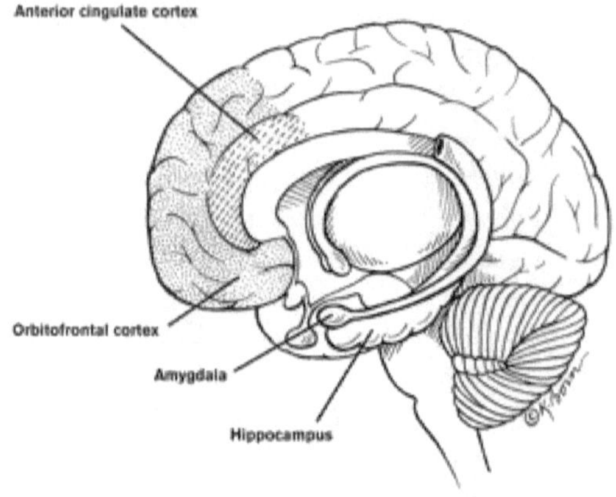

The hippocampus

The hippocampus is a small region of the brain that forms part of the limbic system and is primarily associated with memory and spatial navigation. The hippocampus has a unique shape, similar to that of a horseshoe. It not only assists with the storage of long-term memories but it is also responsible for the memory of the location of objects or people. We would not be able to remember the location of our house if the hippocampus is damaged.
Alzheimer's disease, (a disease that affects elderly people and often results in loss of memory) has been proven to have affected and damaged this area of the brain.

The amygdala (danger detecting brain)
The amygdala is an almond-shaped set of neurons located deep in the brain's medial temporal lobe. When you think of the amygdala, you should think

*of one word" Fear". The amygdala is the reason
we are afraid of things outside our control. It also
controls the way we react to certain stimuli or an
event that causes an emotion that we see as
potentially threatening or dangerous. Conditions
such as anxiety, autism, depression, post-
traumatic stress disorder, and phobias are
suspected of being linked to abnormal functioning
of the amygdala, owing to damage, developmental
problems, or neurotransmitter imbalance.*

The Hypothalamus
*It is a small cone-shaped structure that projects
downward from the brain, ending in the pituitary
(infundibula) stalk, a tubular connection to the
pituitary gland. The hypothalamus contains a
control centre for many functions of the
autonomic nervous system, and it has effects on
the endocrine system because of its complex
interaction with the pituitary gland.
The hypothalamus is mainly responsible for
motivational behaviour. It is the reason we know
when we are hungry or thirsty. The hypothalamus
also helps our body maintain a constant
temperature.
This in brief about how the brain works. Although
I will be introducing many other relevant areas in
the brain as we move on, the detailed explanation
of each and every part of brain described above is
so vast that it is outside the purview of this book.*

The science of fear and memory
Snap judgments are done by spindle-shaped

neurons which respond rapidly are found in abundance in the human brain especially relevant for social relatedness and bonding. These are responsible for us making snap and quick judgments based on the situation as these neurons are relatively thicker and can make high-velocity transmissions.

There are two types of memory stored in our hippocampus, one is implicit and the other is explicit.

Explicit memory is when we try to remember an event or what we ate for dinner yesterday or what was the last movie we saw?

Implicit memory is also known as unconscious memory which reacts with the same emotional events and situations intensively. When the situation is potentially dangerous, it activates the flight, fright freeze response by the amygdala. The alarm system is automatic and before you realise it happens. Thousands of years ago when our ancestors saw a predatory animal like a tiger, it was best for them to react immediately and not think about what to do with the tiger. Thus the repeated conditioning made our amygdala, fast-track the process and kept our ancestors alive. Hence this is a protective response in every individual and saves us when the pathways bypass the frontal lobe and connect to the amygdala.

Now since the amygdala has been conditioned to act in a certain way, the same pathway gets activated when you suddenly hear a noise in a dark room or if there is too much traffic on the road or you are getting late for the interview. Repeated firing of the amygdala for a frivolous situation can create panic attacks and create what we called as stress. Repeated firing strengthens these synapses and increases the strength of the reaction. This is known as chronic stress. It interferes with our decision making and uses a lot of energy. This hinders with our creative thinking, decision making and logical reasoning which are the functions of the prefrontal cortex (PFC). Ideally, the amygdala and occipitofrontal cortex (OFC) should be in harmonious relation with each other. This we call as the learning or calm state. But any emotional surge like fear, anger changes the balance, and amygdale get overactive giving false alarms. This is one of the pathways which act as a hindrance in achieving the right conditions for positive and logical thinking. One more fact of prolonged amygdala stimulation is that it down regulates the receptors on the hippocampus (our memory centre) which makes us difficult to recollect when we are stressed out.

Our autonomic nervous system has two parts that are sympathetic and parasympathetic nervous system. The sympathetic nervous system excites you while the parasympathetic nervous system relaxes you. Accordingly the effects on the heart, blood pressure, metabolism, muscle tension, breathing rate and mental arousal. Accordingly, the amygdala stimulates the sympathetic nervous system which gets the intense effect.

However there is a slight paradox when we avoid what we fear, our fear grows. Initially, our fear does decrease but slowly our anxiety grows. This is followed up by an increase in our fear. For example, when we fear meeting our boss, we avoid to go out for a lunch with him. It may decrease the anxiety for the first time but the next time when we avoid the lunch invitation we increase the anxiety of having a one-on-one

conversation with him.
Procrastination means that you put off things because you think that it is easier on your stress levels. This is one more behaviour pattern associated with prolonged avoidance. You simply build up the anxiety till the last moment and may act in a way which you may regret.

What is neuroplasticity?
Neuroplasticity as the name suggests the brain is like plastic which is bendable. The neuron and their connection can be rewired at any stage in the life unlike the old school of thoughts which believed that the brain is hardwired and cannot undergo change. Also, the new neurons get generated when we learn a new activity or language by releasing Brain Derived Neuroplastic Factor (BDNF). It acts like a fertiliser to make crops grow.
Another interesting fact is about Long-Term Potentiation (LTP) which occurs when excitation between cells is prolonged. This strengthens the connections between the cells and makes them more apt to fire together in the future.

So, to make a summary of the aim of studying the whole science involved in the functioning of the brain is to strengthen our prefrontal lobe and learn how to tame the amygdala. Although the goal sounds very easy in real practice, it's a daunting task to achieve the following. Our thoughts are rigid and hard wired. They are controlled by the emotions and situations we face in our lives. We rarely realise that the brain moves in automation, without our conscious knowledge. The process of automation is so tempting, that our highly charged up a billion *neurons move into a fixed pathway. Any challenge to <u>the</u> system needs a lot of patience and hard work.*

*I have tried to explain these circuits, the related organs and neurochemicals in a lucid and simple way, but in reality, one gets amazed by the speed and complexities of these neuronal circuits. To end the chapter with a glimmer of hope, I want to add the "**brain is more like a plant than a machine**" meaning it is both adaptable and malleable."*

1.

Sam

The degree of attention is directly proportional to the mental force of a thought.

Sam was a bank manager and was working with an international bank for the last 15 years. He had a daughter Anna and a loving wife Jane, who had always been by his side and supported him in his good and bad times. He had a team of co-workers who were ever willing to take up the most difficult tasks in his office under his supervision. Life had been beautiful until recently.

Sam from his college days had great interpersonal skills and would communicate with his friends and fellow students. He was very popular amongst his college mates because of his excellent communicative skills. At times he would mock his beautiful wife, that she wouldn't have noticed him if it weren't for his communication skills. His journey to the bank manager's post was a roller coaster ride and was filled with hardships and difficult times.

There was a moment in his life, where Sam had almost given up on himself because of the unfair and manipulative behaviours of his HR head. He had almost decided to quit, but it was because of Jane, he decided to hold on and trust himself. His HR head didn't like him and would find out the smallest of his mistakes. This had created a sense of self-doubt. He was hesitant in his decisions and would, of-late stammer in his meetings with his clients. Sam knew that the negative feedback was taking a toll on his mind. He knew whatever his HR head was telling him was untrue. It was motivated because of his clout amongst his colleagues. But he simply couldn't stop his mind from thinking because of the negative jibes from him.

It was his wife Jane, who came to his rescue and made him realize that he will be able to overcome these difficult times. She would spend hours with him, reminding him how he used to solve the problems of his friends and relatives in a jiffy. She showed him videos of the speeches, he had delivered in various office, for which he had been praised by one and all. How he was hailed by one and all for his non-judgmental decisions! How they had run away from their house in spite of the opposition from her parents!

Jane couldn't help noticing the mischievous smile on his face. She knew the HR had damaged his self-confidence over a period of time. But she trusted Sam and his ability to bounce back. She knew he will "**Come back**". With all her efforts, Sam started gaining his confidence back and was overlooking the negative comments from the HR and focussed on his work. He would try to logically reason out with him and let go. Sam avoided getting into an unnecessary conversation. As luck and fortune favour the brave, his tormentor was transferred and Sam was back to his usual self again. The incident had convinced him that he was a great fighter and could solve any problem if he had Jane by his side.

But now he was facing a different problem, which even Jane was clueless. His daughter Anna who was 13 years old, a teenager, was obsessed with electronic gadgets. She hardly spoke to anyone in the house, since the last one year and would spend most of her time, either playing on the laptop or chatting with the school friends. Although Jane and Sam were both working parents, they would spend at least two to three hours every day with Anna. But she was obsessed with games, social media and would only reply to them in a few sentences.

Sam and Jane, like most parents realized the need to intervene. They went on a vacation to her favourite place, Switzerland, with the hope that she gets rid of her obsession. But even there, she would be chatting with her friends or playing games. She was disinterested in sightseeing and spending time with the family. This sudden change in their child's behaviour was irritating them.

This change was unacceptable for Sam and he would have arguments with her, when he would tell her to stop using gadgets. Of all the things in life he hated indiscipline and would feel hurt when she back-answered him. This was way beyond his patience levels and he finally decided to put restrictions on the use of gadgets in his daughter's life. Endless chains of arguments between the father-daughter started. This completely shattered the peace and harmony in the family. It became a usual affair when Sam would come from his work, there would be an argument on the dinner table, which would end up with someone sleeping hungry. Jane tried to make both of them understand but deep down her heart, she agreed with what Sam was doing. She was worried about her dropping grades and was scared that this obsession could lead to severe psychological and behaviour problems for Anna in the near future. She knew after speaking to other parents, that this was happenings in most of the houses. Children obsessed with gadgets leading to arguments. But unlike other children, Anna was defiant. Jane could not let her child destroy herself and would try to explain her most of the times. But even her patience was running out.

This was going on for quite a while, until one fine day, Anna suddenly ran away from the house. They tried to find her everywhere, but she was not to be located. They found a note in her room saying "Papa and Mama, if you have so much of a problem with me and my ways of life, it is best that I leave the house, so you and I can live in peace." Sam panicked and went to his friend Joe, the Sergeant and registered a missing complaint. They sent out search parties to locate her. Sam felt the same sinking feeling which he had felt years back, only to find that his wife Jane, was not in a state to support him. Actually, he was more worried, that she doesn't get a nervous breakdown. It was making him feel really lonely and scared, as he started worrying about all the negative things which could have happened. It was two days and she was nowhere to be found. He started worrying about, how she will survive as she did not have any money. On the other side, Jane was crying, and had stopped eating food for the last two days. He felt drained, and was short of ideas on how to find her. The fear of her being in trouble, and the guilt of being too strict with her, was making it impossible for him to sleep even for a second. He was known as a "problem solver," and now he was getting stuck. He had always helped people in more grave and difficult circumstances, but why was he unable to rescue his family from this dreadful event. He needed to speak to someone.

Our brain is highly neuroplastic in nature and we have already discussed this in the chapter on science. But there is one more quality of our brain. The brain is lazy in nature. Especially, as we grow up, it doesn't like to work hard. If the brain is lazy, then how can we perform these complex tasks and deal with complicated situations? How can we come with so many ideas and thoughts in our workplace or personal lives? Also, the brain is constantly functioning throughout the day. Approximately we have 60000 thoughts in a span of 24 hours. There are 86400 seconds in 24 hours and we sleep for 8 hours a day. So eventually we have a single thought, every second, which is a lot of work. Let me come back to the statement that "the brain is lazy." The effort the brain takes to repeat thoughts is negligible to the one it takes, to come with a new thought or an idea. Hence, what we think in the day, are more repeated thoughts or thoughts linked to each other. Let me give you an example. Say in the morning if I decide, I am going to my clinic. The next thought will be, which patient has an appointment today? Will he come on time? If he is my old patient, then, would his ailment have been cured and so on? If you go to see, the brain has processed the same basic thought, but related it to another event and repeated the thought in various ways.
Another function of the brain, is that it stores the information it perceives in the form of images. Most of the new information it stores, is related to a previous image and so on. This is responsible for having different perceptions of the same

image. This is happening at such a tremendous speed, that for us, to comprehend and analyse, why or what is happening, our brain has already executed the thought. But the effort it takes to come up with a new idea or thought, is tremendous and it lazily relates to the old image and thought processes. The time taken is so swift that we do not get time, to actually reflect on the thoughts. You can say that "the brain tricks us into it". However, there is no intention behind it. Our brain follows the old pattern much easier as compared to forming a new thought. Say for instance, if I am going to my clinic, I can appreciate the beauty of a seashore next to my house or check out the effort of the traffic police doing his job. Hearing the birds sing or chirping of kids going to school. All this will need an extra effort for my brain to process. And our brain doesn't put in that effort and hence behaves lazily. So, it needs that extra force to make it work more effectively and come with new ideas or in layman's terms "out of the box" or innovative solutions or ideas.

*Another interesting thing about our brain, is that it tends to be more inclined to this old pattern, which forms our perception. It gets entangled unknowingly, using our cognitive functions in prefrontal lobe and parietal lobes. So, even if it does put minimal effort, it ends up being less productive, in terms of actual problem-solving. This is one of the reasons why the brain is also called **"a creator of its own problem"**. In spite of having a highly efficient prefrontal lobe or the thinking brain, we find ourselves getting entangled in complex but solvable situations in our lives.*

In physics, a force or effort is any interaction

that, when unopposed, will change the motion of an object. A force can cause an object with mass to change its velocity (which

includes to begin moving from a state of rest), i.e., to accelerate. A force can be defined as a push or a pull, which acts upon an object as a result of its interaction with another object. When one object exerts a force on another object, it always experiences, an equal opposing force in return from the object, it exerted the force on.

The word force is used for countable objects and effort for uncountable objects. Thoughts and ideas are uncountable, so effort used by the brain, has to overcome the inertia by the old pathways, which act as an opposing force and a hindrance in forming new pathways.

Newton's second law of motion can be formally stated, the acceleration of an object, as produced by a net force, is directly proportional to the magnitude of the net force, in the same direction as the net force, and inversely proportional to the mass of the object. Here again, the force of our thought is directly proportional to the magnitude of the attention over it and is inversely proportional to the inertia by the old pathways and the lazy property of the brain.

The next question in our mind is if the brain is lazy and follows a definite pattern than how did mankind come up with path-breaking ideas and have come with great innovate solutions. There has to be something in the same brain, which must be creating enough force to overcome these rigid and fixed pathways and untangle the thought process. When we are in a complex situation and are short of ideas or solutions, we have two options, either we stop thinking about them or we get entangled in the thought process.

The chances that the solution we get in the latter situation is less and at times distressing as compared to letting go of the thought, and tackle the situation later on. The brain tends to opt out rather than going through the distress .Every year on 1st January millions of people make resolutions for the New Year, but very few of them, actually follows them. But I can guarantee that most of them, believe that they will be benefited by following the resolution, if they have it within their control. People usually say that they do not have adequate belief and hence do not follow their resolutions or decisions. But they all accept that if they do, they will gain.

Attention *is the ability of the brain to selectively concentrate on one aspect of the environment while ignoring other things. There are two types of attention in two separate regions of the brain. The prefrontal cortex (directly behind the forehead) is in charge of wilful concentration. If you are studying for a test or writing a novel, the impetus and the orders come from the PFC.*

But if there is a sudden, riveting event - the attack of a tiger or the scream of a child - it is the parietal cortex (behind the ear) that is activated. Scientists have learned that these two brain regions sustain concentration when the neurons emit pulses of electricity at specific rates - faster frequencies for the automatic processing of the parietal region, slower frequencies for the deliberate, intentional work of the prefrontal region.

During the twentieth century, researchers developed a better understanding of what it really means to pay attention. A few key developments include:

1920s: A Russian scientist named Ivan Petrovich

Pavlov observed some of the physical signs of attention in dogs and other animals, which came to be known as the orienting response. These signs included pricked-up ears, turning the head toward the stimulus, increased muscle tension, and other changes in the body. In his most famous experiment, Pavlov found that he could train dogs to associate the ringing of a bell with the delivery of food. Pavlov's discovery gave rise to a school of psychology known as behaviourism, which studies how behaviour is caused by the brain's responses to external factors.

1950s: The theory of the bottleneck is used to describe the process of attention. Scientists theorise that the many signals entering the central nervous system are placed in temporary storage and then are analysed for their importance. In this way, a person can filter out what needs attention and only allow those signals to pass through for further processing in the brain.

1990s: The development of new scanning technologies such as positron emission tomography and magnetic resonance imaging allows researchers to watch the brain in action. For example, researchers at Duke University in North Carolina recently used an MRI scanner to take 480 snapshots per minute of the brain activity of several volunteers as they watched a computer-controlled television screen. The scans showed how areas of activity in the brain shift as the person shift attention. Many other studies have used this technology to determine how different areas of the brain are involved in different activities.

This is an overly simplified explanation of a complex process. There are other parts of the brain and nervous system that play a role in the process of paying attention. For example, a group of structures in the middle of the brain compose the limbic system, which is linked to various emotions and feelings such as fear, pleasure, and sadness.

There is a group of Neuroscientists who believe that attention is largely a function of the brain's reticular activating system or RAS. This system includes a group of nerve fibres located in several parts of the brain, including the thalamus, hypothalamus, brainstem and cerebral cortex. The RAS seems to account for the shifts in people's level of involvement with their surroundings, which ranges anywhere from full attention to sleep. When the system is fully operating, a person is awake, alert, and attentive; this would be the case when a person is listening to an interesting lecture or taking an important test. When the RAS is less active, a person is tired or inattentive. The highway signs urging drivers to "Stay Awake - Take a Break" actually are related to the RAS; it is much more difficult for people to pay attention when they are tired. Within the RAS, the thalamus appears to play a key role in the moment-to-moment changes in the focus of attention. The thalami and cerebral cortex cooperate to register any incoming sensory signals, evaluate their contents, and mobilise brain resources in response to the demands made. Put simply, the thalami receive the messages that come through a person's senses and then relay the information to the proper receiving areas in the brain.

These structures are thought to play some role in how people decide to focus their attention.

For example, when a student sits at a desk to read a school textbook, a variety of complex emotions may play a role in her decision to focus on the text: pleasure in the subject matter, fear of doing poorly on the next test, desire to perform well during class discussion, and so forth. To focus in on the task at hand, she must tune out all other stimuli, such as the other books scattered around the room, the sound of children playing outside, the colour of the desk pad, and the ticking of the clock.

Attention is not always under a person's control, however. If someone comes bursting into the room or turns on a stereo at full volume, the student's attention would likely be drawn away from the book. Thus, attention may be captured by an unexpected event rather than voluntarily directed toward it.

The brain requires to overcome the inertia and the magnitude of force or effort of thought and make a decision and then to sustain the newly created force of the new idea to have the desired result. We also term this as the perseverance of an act.

Attention is required for any new thought to initiate which we call it as decision making. When we make a decision a certain amount of attention is always required. This does not necessarily convert into a tangible action if the attention on the thought is not adequate. Over a period of time, many of our decisions which may seem to be a highly powerful and strong die a natural death. The reason behind this is that the attention while making the decision was inadequate and so was the force generated. Also when the necessary actions were initiated on the thought the attention was diverted to something more important at that moment.

The sustainability of the attention and the continuous stimulation of the pathways and structure becomes a very big determinant of the successful implementation of any decision. This is evident when we decide on something, but we do not put adequate attention on it to follow it up and bring it to its logical conclusions. Of course, there are other emotional turmoil's and distractions in everybody's life. But when we want to increase the mental force of a thought or idea, it needs to be given maximum attention by shutting off the inputs from other sources. This mental force, thus created has the maximum probability to reach its desired goal.

The degree of attention is directly proportional to the mental force of a thought.

Sam was in a state of shock and guilt because he never expected Anna to take such an extreme step. He wasn't prepared for this. Although he was able to help everyone in their difficult times, his amygdala (the emotional brain) was firing and this was freezing his thought process. This is common when we are in a stressful situation. Our logical thinking suddenly gets stuck and we find it difficult to make the right decision. His worries were compounded by Jane's condition, like in most of the situations in our life, where we have to deal with multiple problems at the same time.

Our brain also has a negative bias which in turn very conveniently connects all information and interpret negative consequences for every problem when it is under stress. Say, if we have a bad day, we start getting annoyed with situations, which were not as irritating in our regular life, as we feel at that moment. Awareness of the process of thinking decreases our sufferings and we are able to come back into the right state of mind early. There is always a lag time for everyone but the time taken to bounce back varies. This can be greatly enhanced by focusing on our problem, filtering out the distraction and solving the issues one at a time.

So Sam needed to focus on his problem and try to block all the distractions in his life. He needed to tackle one situation at a time and this was possible only if he was by himself. Many people take the help of their friends to resolve their problem but the most relevant advice always comes from within. Sam's mind was overactive, like in most of us, in stressful situations, with the brain firing multiple solutions. He needed to choose the right decision, without being too judgmental. He had to focus on his problem and gather more information. Only then he would be able to come up with the best solution. At times there are multiple stages in a solution. It is better we focus on the events and make the most appropriate decision with a series of alternative solutions. This is only possible when we increase the attention to the problem.

However, the chances of making the right decision increase multi fold when there is adequate attention given to the problem and the probability of the outcome are directly proportional to the belief in the decision (the force of the thought).

Sam in spite of searching for two days, he was unable to find his daughter Anna. On the other

side, his wife Jane was deteriorating. He realised
that he needs to act fast as his wife was
inconsolable. Also, he needs to get Anna back
before she endangers her life. He decided to go
away from his house for a day and stay in a hotel.
It seemed cruel to Jane, as he was leaving her
alone in the midst of this difficult time. He knew
he had to do it, as he had to come up with a
solution. He could not let his family perish with
this incident.

He arranged for his sister to come and stay the
next day. He sat down in the hotel room thinking
about what he would have advised his friend if he
would have been in a similar situation.

It looked rather funny, but he would sit down on
one chair pretending, he was Sam and sit on the
other chair answering as if he was the friend in
trouble. As he repeated this act, he would jot
down relevant points.

He started writing down the mobile numbers of
her friends and started calling them up once
again. This time he inquired in detail about her
behaviour in school in the last few days,
frantically trying to find a clue. He tried hard not
to feel guilty, about the fact that he had put
restrictions on her. On inquiring he learned that
Anna talked to a boy Jonathan in her class for
hours together during lunch breaks and after
school. At times they sat down for a couple of
hours after school, chatting in solitaire, on the
pretext of going for tuitions. He realised that this
was the missing clue which he must follow up.
He had the gut feeling that Jonathan would be
knowing about her whereabouts. He tried hard not
to get carried away with his emotions and headed
straight to his house. He was greeted by his
mother who seemed to be a nice lady. Luckily

Jonathan had just come back from his tuitions and Sam informed him that Anna was missing and whether he knew about her whereabouts. Jonathan said he had not seen her in school for last two days. Sam had an urge to really smack this guy, as he was convinced that he knew where Anna was. He tried to not let his parenteral anguish come in between his search to find out where Anna was. He asked him if he had observed any change in her behaviour or what conversation they had in the last few days. He learned Anna was in touch with guys from neighbouring street, who were involved in drugs. Anna used to spend a lot of time with them and would chat with them for hours together on phone. These guys were a bunch dropouts who stayed in a rented flat and used to work during the daytime and party at night. Jonathan had tried his best to convince her to avoid their company as they would get her in trouble someday. However, he had never seen Anna taking drugs. He tried to convince her not to hang out with those guys but she wouldn't listen. He gave Sam the address of those boys.

Sam's fears multiplied on hearing about the school dropouts and drugs. His amygdala sent signals that his daughter was in a grave and dangerous situation and he had to try to rescue her before she gets into trouble. Still, his prefrontal lobe (the thinking brain) wanted him not to prejudge and try to locate his daughter first. He also felt the same guilt again, but only this time it was because he had judged Jonathan too early. He went to the address which Jonathan had given him, determined to find his daughter and get her back. He was ready to deal with any situation. Even if the guys had guns he would get his daughter back. Somewhere deep in his mind, there was a fear that his daughter might have been kidnapped or even worse. He knocked at the door and a boy of around 21 years opened the door. He asked Sam who he was and what did he want? Sam told him he was Sam and was looking for his daughter who had not come home for two days. The boy immediately answered, "Are you Anna's father?" Suddenly, blood rushed to Sam's face and eyes were red. He controlled his anger and said, "Yes, yes. How do you know Anna? Where is my daughter? I hope you have not harmed her. Otherwise, you are in deep trouble." The boy put his hand on Sam's shoulder and told him, "Relax sir". He shouted loudly "Anna! Could you come down for a moment?" He told Sam that they have been trying to ask Anna for the last two days where she stays but she had not been answering. It was great that Sam had come down so he could speak to her, as she was not eating food and was not talking to anyone. The boy's tone was gentle. Anna came down and saw Sam. She lost her mind at the boys and yelled at him, "Why did you not tell me that it was my father?" Sam apologised to Anna for his behaviour and sat with her trying to understand what the real problem was. Why did she leave the house and why was she behaving so irrational? He learned that Anna had broken up with her boyfriend 6 months back and he was blackmailing her for the last 6 months with some photographs he had captured without her knowledge. She tried to tell him a couple of times, but most of the times she was scared as he would get angry. She knew Sam was conservative and didn't like her having any boyfriends. These guys were helping her to trap him and they succeeded in getting the photographs, only to

know that there were duplicate copies. The boy
was extorting money from her which she had
borrowed from these guys. Sam told her that he
was not angry with her and hugged her. He
apologised to her for not understanding her. He
said he would talk to his sergeant friend who
would solve the problem. He thanked the boys for
all the help they had given Anna. He apologised
to the boy who opened the door for being
judgmental about him and talking to him rudely.
Jane was ecstatic when she saw Anna. Her
boyfriend was located and was arrested and all the
photographs and negatives were recovered after a
few days.
As the family was sitting on the lawn with Jane
cuddling in her husband's lap. Jane winked at him
and exclaimed, "Sam, Mr. Problem Solver, what a
comeback!" He realised he needed to pay more
attention to his family

2.

Tom

Minds like other planets and organism tends to function in automation. It is the level of awareness that enables us to break these automations and make conscious and path-breaking decisions...

Sam was extremely happy that he had successfully got his daughter safely back home. He had understood her problems and found out the necessary resolutions. Like any father, Sam was proud of his achievement and delighted he had got his daughter back home safely. Jane and he decided to throw a party and invite all their friends and share their happiness. He also wanted to invite his school mates whom he had not met for a long time.

So he called up his school friend, Tom who was a software engineer and was once his close friend. Sam hadn't spoken to him after passing out from school, so he decided to give him a call and invite him to the party. Tom readily accepted his invitation. Sam was shocked by Tom's transition as he was a shy and reserved child in school and would rarely mix up with other kids. Now he was sounding confident and positive.

Tom was reared with a lot of financial hardships faced by his parents. In his early days, Tom stayed in a rented place and used to wear borrowed clothes. Only when he reached college that the family was able to afford some luxury. Right from the early years, he had understood the value of earning money. He had learned the lessons of budgeting and suppressing desires and cravings from his early childhood. In spite of his parents trying their level best, they were finding it difficult to make the ends meet. Those were the days of recession and eating in restaurants was once in a year episode in Tom's family. Every toy Tom had ever played, was either donated by some family friend or bought at a clearance sale. One could say Tom had lived with an inferiority complex, until he was 14 and then his father had his share of luck. His father started a business which gave good profits and they were able to shift to a house of their own. Tom used to do many house jobs like cleaning cars or babysitting from the age of 10. He wanted to help his father. He was a disciplined and a good boy and was always loved by everyone. Tom was a quiet child and used to generally avoid engaging with people. At times, Tom avoided conversations because he feared that he would be teased for his borrowed clothes and used toys. It was rare to see him getting agitated or angry. He was a hardworking and dedicated boy and these were the qualities which always got him high grades in school. Sam always liked him because he would help him to learn difficult lessons and he would, in turn, share his lunch with him. Sam frequently called him to his house to play with his new television games which were a big hit in those times. Tom used to avoid reacting to his classmates who were teasing him because of his old school uniform. Sam was always by his side and would at times fight for him. Since Tom had a habit of suppressing his emotions in public, he would rarely react to any provocation. Once, one of his class fellow students had hidden the teacher book and broken her chair. The teacher fell down and had a fracture on her hand. The group of mischievous boys blamed Tom for the mischief. Tom knew who had played the prank. But he was unable to gather the courage, to tell the truth. It was Sam who came to his rescue and saved him from being expelled from the school. He was often bullied by his school and college friends because of his meek behaviour. However, all this did not stop him from excelling in his academics and he was always in the merit list. He was praised by one and all for his hard work and dedication.

He cleared his engineering college with high grades and was hired immediately. He was praised by his bosses for his dedication and loyalty and got his promotions much faster than others. This made his colleagues jealous and envious of him. He was married to an English teacher Susan, who was a very calm lady. She used to spend a lot of her time doing social service as she believed in compassion and empathy for all. They had a son by the name Gavin, who was 7 years and was an extremely obedient child. Susan used to tease Tom that her son was a carbon copy of him but Tom use to feel upset whenever she said that. He would always reply **"Make him like you so I can love him more."**

It was a Saturday, Tom's boss called him in his cabin for an urgent work. This was the very first time Tom was ever called personally in a face to face meeting with The CEO of his firm except during his interview. He was scared as there were rumours of that the company was planning to lay off the non-performers. It was a common strategy in a company those days, due to the recession to lay off their employees so as to reduce the cost. He went to his boss's cabin. With cold feet and hands shaking, he knocked on the CEO's cabin. A voice from inside called him, "Come in". Tom entered the room and was surprised to find the president and vice president seated in the room. He realised the "D-day" had come, which he had been ruminating about, since the last week. The moment of truth had come. How will he tell Susan about this? The home loan was due in a week, Tom wondered how he would manage to payback the loans. The CEO started, "Tom, You have been reading in the newspaper about the recession and how companies are laying off their employees. No company does this by choice, but there are situations where such hard decisions have to be made. This is the most difficult job, I hate doing. So, I want to tell you, that there is a good news and a bad news. Which news would you like to hear first?" The CEO asked with a wicked smile on his face like the Devil asking you for your soul. Tom's heart sank and he was almost in tears. He had always found it difficult to engage in an intense and difficult situation. However, he had to answer. With a heavy heart, he said, "Please give me the bad news first". "Well, Tom since you insist I will tell you the bad news first. It has been decided that the company's production Manager 'Smith' will have to go. He has not been as efficient and productive as the company expected him to be. His contract will be terminated from tomorrow and he will have to vacate the office by tomorrow. The company can no longer continue with such irresponsible and lazy employees anymore". By now Tom was almost going to faint. Smith and he were great friends and it was Smith who had recommended him for the present job in the company. Tom could feel a current of fear running down the spine because the next person could be him." He was not as experienced and talented as Smith and why would the company keep him in difficult times? Why was the CEO telling him all this? What could be so good about being fired?" he thought. Fear was converted into anger as he realized the insensitivity of the CEO. However, he suppressed his emotions as always and mumbled," What is the good news"." Glad you asked", the CEO replied, "You have been promoted as the production manager with a team of 250 odd engineers under you. That is the good news." Tom was shocked, appalled, surprised, astonished, dumbfounded….. You name the emotion! He was feeling it at that moment. It took him time to absorb good news. The CEO offered him a chair and a glass of water. Everyone in the room congratulated him. "But there are few jobs you need to do first. You need to go tell Smith about this and you need to address your team about this news and how you plan to move forward with your new job profile. My only advice to you is that until today, you could always do your job meticulously but now you need to engage with your team and make them work in the same way. You need to think about this and the company believes you would be a wonderful Production manager." Tom's happiness knew no bounds. He wanted to call up Susan and tell her the good news. But he wasn't sure how to tell Smith about the bad news. He went to his table and sat for a minute thinking about how to tell Smith, about that the management's decision and he was given his chair. Smith would feel cheated. He gathered courage and went straight to Smith's cabin, which was going to be his cabin soon. He told Smith that the management wanted him to quit and he had been told to give this message to him. Smith was surprisingly calm and he told him that he expected this to happen. He also knew through sources that Tom was given his post. He warned Tom that it wasn't easy dealing with the team as they were the ones who were responsible for getting him in this awkward situation. He wished him all the best and told him that he would pray for him. This behaviour perplexed Tom as he couldn't understand how somebody could be so calm, when he is laid off. There was a sign of relief on Smith's face, which Tom recollected as he went back to his cabin. This scared him all the more. But he was so preoccupied with the good news of his promotion, that he called up Susan and informed her about it. The next two days Tom and Susan had a great time celebrating his success. What they didn't realise was the reason behind the sigh of relief Smith had on that day.

Like the CEO had told Tom, he had called up his team of engineers in the coming weekend. He was prepared to have a fruitful and motivating talk with the team. He sat up late at night and got his speech ready. He wore the new overcoat which Susan had got the previous day as he believed that the first impression would be the last impression. He wanted to impress his team. He reached the meeting hall which had roughly around 150 engineers from various branches. Although he knew some of them, most of the people were strangers as they were from other branches.

Rover, Solomon, and Gasparov were the Assistant

Managers who waited for him at the door. They gave him a bouquet of flowers and took him to the stage. Rover started the speech by greeting Tom and introducing him to the audience. As Tom was getting up to start his speech, Rover continued. "Bootlicking and not talent is the order of the day in most companies". He also hurled many indirect insults over Tom's inexperience which made Tom feel uncomfortable. Same was the case with Gasporav who was next to introduce him. He wished Tom luck and hoped that he would be able to survive as the production manager until Christmas that year. These comments were met with a lot of cheer from the crowd. Tom was unsettled and did not know how to react. He suppressed his anxiety and went to the podium for delivering his speech. Just then the smile of Smith came to his mind. How he had wished, he would have discussed at length with Smith about these assistant managers, so he would be better prepared to face this unexpected turn of events. He started his speech, but there was a lot of booing mixed with sarcastic laughter. He couldn't believe he was dealing with a bunch of well-educated adults, behaving like rowdy teenagers. One of the gentlemen got up and told Tom to go home, as he was incapable and lacked basic experience. Tom tried in vain to get the colleagues to behave soberly. "At least listen to me first and then decide whether I am worth it or not", he kept on yelling to an unruly crowd. All three Rover, Gasparov and Solomon were inciting the crowd. The crowd started chanting "Down with Tom". Tom started losing his patience. Unable to control his emotion, he threw the mike at the crowd and walked out. He went straight to his cabin and rushed to meet the CEO. The CEO asked him," What was the matter? Why was it so urgent to meet him without informing the secretary?" Tom apologized and narrated the incident to him, which he listened intently. He asked Tom" Why did you have to throw the mike and walk away? You could have dealt with the situation more maturely". He also pointed out that three in charge were highly influential and popular amongst the other employees so it was impossible to fire them in the present situation. Smith had a similar problem and that cost him his job. He should learn how to deal with them or quit the job. As for the rest of the crowd, all the engineers were extremely talented but misguided. It is the job of the production manager to get the house in order. If Tom was unable to deal with them, he had no choice but to hire a capable person for the job. He gave Tom two weeks and report to him with the three of them by his side or start looking for another job. He believed in Tom's ability but Tom had to deliver.

Tom's dreams were demolished. His worst fears had come true. He was scared and the same fear which has been in his mind for so many years had suddenly blown out of proportions. His habit of holding back his emotions, was creating a complete breakdown of his thinking process. He had reduced his diet, hardly spoke to anyone in the house. This change in behaviour got Susan worried. She decided to take the matters in her hand and forced him to take leave for a couple of days. She, along with Tom went for a small vacation where Tom finally told him about the meetings and conversation he had with the CEO. Susan listened to him empathetically and saw her husband speak out all the fears and emotional turmoil. Tom had never spoken about them to anyone and had kept to himself for all these years. Tom wept like a small child as he narrated the incidents in his childhood and how he could not gather courage even if he wanted to. They stayed up the entire night with Susan listening to her husband's ordeal and how helpless he was in his past and present life. She understood why it was hard for him to take on the unruly staff who were actually simply revolting to the company policy and had nothing to do with him.

Automation is defined as the technique, method, or system of operating or controlling a process by highly automatic means, as by electronic devices, reducing human intervention to a minimum.
To simplify it further it is the method of making a machine, a process, or a system work without being directly controlled by a person.
Automation represents one of the major trends of the 20th century. The drive to provide increased levels of control of electro-mechanical systems, and with it, a corresponding distancing of the human from direct system control has grown out of the belief that automated systems provide superior reliability, improved performance and reduced costs for the performance of many functions.
Similarly, we have the universe and nature around us, working in automation. Let me try to explain this in detail. The planets revolve around the sun and the satellites (the moon revolves around the earth in automation). Although it is not absolute because there are instances where the balance between them changes, what we know as variations in the gravitational force causing storms and cyclones. In physics, Gravitational

force and the electromagnetic quantum dynamics are two principles to explain why the organism and the universe move in automation.

But the majority of the time, the universe tends to move in automation. Similarly, the life cycles of organisms on planet earth move in automation. Nobody can deny the fact that we are born, then we get young, turn old and finally die. These are the facts which we have to live with every single day of our life. The heart beats every single moment, the breath and the various organs like liver makes bile or the kidneys making urine, they all move in automation without any voluntary control.

But there are instances when this automation is momentarily disturbed, which changes the balance. So as in an infectious disease or neoplasms or any other disease once the automation is broken, it rewires and starts moving into other automation, only this time it destroys the body rather than being in harmony. We call this a parasitic relationship rather than symbiotic. When we intervene with treatment in the form of medicines or therapy, we break this automation and try to get the body back to harmony or homeostasis.

The fact that the universe and all its beings are moving in automation is now well established. There are subtle moments which change this automation to make them move into new automation. For example comets or meteors changing the path.

Similarly, our brain and its pathways tend to automate. This has resulted in us making those micro and macro changes in the brain when we learn to ride a bicycle or a motorbike. Initially, when we learn to ride a bicycle we all have had fallen off balance at some moment. Once we have learned and the brain pathways have become autonomous, we do not necessarily get off balance easily and fall off the bicycle. Even when we are talking to someone while riding we are able to maintain the balance. But during our learning, we need to have maximum awareness and focus on the task, be it learning how to read and write or riding a bicycle. It can be learning how to communicate or the social interactions in early childhood. Our awareness is at its maximum. But once the learning is done, the brain and its pathway set the same task into automation.

Since the ancient history of mankind, reacting to a stressful situation or managing difficult emotions are some of the things has always been understated and not given its due importance. But today in this fast-paced world, managing thoughts and emotions has become one of the most essential skills. Multinational companies are on a lookout for such employees having high emotional quotient who can challenge this automation.

In many cases, automation has provided the desired benefits and has extended system functionality well beyond existing human capabilities. Along with these benefits, however, a certain price has been extracted.

In 1989, a US Air B-737 failed to take-off at New York's LaGuardia Airport, landing in the nearby river (National Transportation Safety Board, 1990). The precipitating cause was an accidental disarming of the auto throttle. Neither the captain nor the first officer monitored the critical flight parameters in order to detect and correct the problem, thus the take-off was not aborted in a timely manner, resulting in the loss of the aircraft and two passengers.

In 1983, a Korean Airlines flight was shot down over the (then) USSR with no survivors. The aircraft was interpreted as hostile when it travelled into Soviet airspace without authorisation or radio contact. Although the critical equipment was never recovered, it is believed that an erroneous entry was made into the flight navigation system early in the flight (Stein, 1983). The crew unknowingly flew to the wrong coordinates, rely on the automated system and unaware of the error.

In each of these cases, the human operators overseeing the automated systems were unaware of the critical features of the systems they were operating. They were unaware of the state of the automated system and were unaware of the aircraft parameters the automation was responsible for.

Originally situation awareness was a term used in the aircraft pilot community. This has developed a major concern in many other domains where people operate complex, dynamic systems, including the nuclear power industry, automobiles, air traffic control, medical systems, teleoperations, maintenance, and advanced manufacturing systems.

Achieving situation awareness is one of the most challenging aspects of these operators' jobs and is central to good decision making and performance.

One thing is absolutely clear that awareness can break this automation formed in the brain pathway. When the brain works in automation, the receptors of the synapses in the neural pathway get primed to the neurotransmitter released. Repetitive stimulation of these pathways strengthens the circuit. Hence in times of emotional turmoil or stress, the brain chooses the more fixed and rigid path and you have a very little say in what choice you make in the given situation. Hence, in a complex or difficult situation, you cannot think of an alternative or what is known as lateral thinking. Out of the box thinking is another fine example of awareness, breaking the automatons of the mind. Repeated conditioning with years of repeated firing of the neural paths makes them work without any regulations and in automation. It has been through various studies that the amount awareness, we bring into any automation, especially through mindfulness practice when we start observing our heartbeats or breath, we are able to manage emotional turmoil and volatile situations. Significant changes in the prefrontal lobes of monks are seen who have a practice mindfulness meditation of 10000 hours or more. They are also less reactive to highly violent or charged up visual stimuli. This awareness helps us to insulate the negative or disturbing thoughts and focus on the task at hand. The higher the awareness levels the more the mind can challenge this automation.

Insights

Tom from birth had a habit of suppressing his emotions. He had been doing this right from his childhood days. He was a hardworking person, but he never stood up for what he thought. Tom would give in to other people's manipulation. This was happening so often that he lost his confidence to confront his tormentors. Many people build a wall around them when they can hide in safety. Some start blaming their destiny and go into a defensive state of mind. We get driven into fixed thinking in a crisis situation, like in Tom's case, suppressing his emotions without actually realising it. This is termed as automation of thought processes. All this was happening because the thought processes have gone into an automation and there is no active thinking happening to resolve the problem.

Also, not everyone is bold enough to confront an uncomfortable situation head on and hence, get driven into reacting to the situation. Tom was so much agitated that he threw the mike without actually realising that by doing, so he was accepting his failure to deal with the situation. It is common to be agitated because of sudden change of events but resilient people come back and deal with the situation more naturally. Tom told Susan about every situation in his life, when he had suppressed his mind from reacting. It has been observed that when we let out anger, our sufferings increase. When we let out our sorrow or share our grief we give space to new thoughts and have a higher chance of coming up with a resolution.

The more we are aware of the automation, like in Tom's case, where he was suppressing his emotions, we are in a better position to overcome this automation of thought processes, formed in our mind. It is not always easy to overcome most of these fixed automated thoughts but in extreme situations, people have come up with breakthrough ideas and overcome their shortcomings. This has been true for many successful people around us. Hence, every extreme situation always presents us with the possibility of coming up with an opportunity

So coming back to Tom and the changes in his work profile. Susan had understood after listening to her husband compassionately. The only advice she gave him, was that she believed in him and supported any decision he will take in the future. She believed that he was the most deserving person to be the production manager, as stated by her seniors. He had the qualities suited for the job, which very few have. He needs to believe in them for getting the answer to his problem. She or any other human was not capable of resolving the issue. Tom was very relieved after speaking out his mind out to Susan. He was reassured by Susan's statements that she was not judging him. He never understood why he was promoted in the first place as he never was so good with his interpersonal skills. So he started listing down all his strengths and weaknesses in his behaviour. Tom realised he was a hardworking and focused employee. He rarely interfered in people's matters and was the last one to poke his head into others issues. He realised in the given scenario, the management wanted a calm guy, who did not get involved in unnecessary arguments. They wanted an employee who would stand as a role model for others to follow. The next thing Tom realised his biggest weakness was engaging in difficult conversations, especially where people would challenge or make fun of him. He also realized that the employees were trying to tell him something if overlooked their unruly behaviour. He needed to communicate with them separately and try to find out what they wanted to say. He suddenly felt a wave of confidence and his face was beaming with new hope, like an employee on the first day of his job. The very first thing he did when he re-joined, he went to Solomon, Rover and Gasparov's desk and met them individually. Of course, they were surprised at the production manager's visit. They tried to mock him, but Tom was as cool as a cucumber. He told them he had gone through their track records and was highly impressed. He praised their efficient working style and how the company had benefitted because of their brilliant communication skills. He realised that the three of them were due for a promotion. He would recommend them for a promotion. He surprised all of them by telling them this.

Tom had realized that they had provoked the rest of the engineers and would keep finding faults in the way companies manage their employees. This was all happening because of management's decision not to promote them since last 3 years. Having understood the problem the next would be how to pacify them. He had already gone through their profiles and each of them was individually, very talented. He had got an insight into how to solve the problem. He straight went to the CEO's office and requested him to hold a party for the engineers on the weekend and this time he wanted to call their family. The CEO was surprised at this request by Tom, but he knew he had to give him a fair chance, after what had happened in Tom's last interaction with the engineers.

Tom had prepared a powerful presentation after interviewing many of the engineers in his cabin. He spends three days to get the presentation up to the mark for the party. Tom with his tuxedo and his beautiful wife Susan by his side reached the venue. His heartbeat skipped as the vision of the previous episode flashed through his mind. The presentation started in the same way like the previous episode with Gasparov and Solomon determined to embarrass and prove a point to the management. They wanted the management to realise that it was not easy to deal with such a huge number of educated skilled engineers. They did not buy Tom's gesture of promotion. Gasparov started introducing Tom when Tom suddenly got up and took over the mike. He excused himself and apologised to everyone for his behaviour last time. He even joked about how he felt on the stage last time and was in two minds to wear a helmet for his speech today. He told Gasporav that he would not let any of three speak today as this was their day. Tom said he was told by the management to honour their most efficient employees and he was given the job to do this. In his video presentation, he showed slide after slide how the employees appreciated the good work done by the three of them. Tom told the gathering that the management could not decide whom to make the production manager as the three of them were equally talented and hence they decided to appoint him. He acknowledged their efforts and sacrifice of the family of engineers, which had grown the company to this level. He expected each and every engineer to grow and make the company reach greater heights like the three of them. He recognised that he was very lucky to have such a great team and was honoured to be their production manager. He called families of Solomon, Gasporav, and Rover on stage and honoured them. The whole hall resonated loudly with claps and cheers, making Susan realized that her husband had transformed from a caterpillar into a butterfly. The three assistant managers were spellbound and overwhelmed by the appreciation of their new boss. Gasparov hugged Tom and whispered in his ears, "I am sorry". Tom with a smile on his face told him "Thank you if it weren't for the three of you, he never could realise what a great team he had". The rest of the party went smoothly. Tom couldn't help noticing the smiles on the face of his three assistant managers. He knew the time had come for making the next move.

The next day he told his secretary to call the three assistant managers for an urgent meeting. He had already spoken to the CEO about promoting three employees from the pool of engineers to the post of special managers as he would be able to work more efficiently. He called up the secretary to make a list of probable for the post of special managers and schedule a meeting in the next few days. Gasparov, Solomon, and Rover entered his office. Tom greeted them and told them that a new assignment has been given by the management and he expected them to form groups and submit the project at the earliest. He couldn't trust anyone with this as he was busy with recruiting new assistant managers and reducing their workload. He had convinced the management that all the important projects be handled by them and recruit new special managers for the routine projects. He wanted all of them to get their dues so he wanted them to use their resources and give the best outcome. The three of them agreed to live up to his expectations and not let him down. As they started leaving Gasparov told Solomon," Finally somebody has come who realised our hard work and efforts." Tom was happy as the body language of the three of them was positive. He spoke to all the new probable for the post of special managers and zeroed them to the three most suited for the job. He went to the CEOs cabin with the list and told him he plans to give them all the major projects to the three of them and train them in the next six months. "What about the existing Assistant managers", the CEO interrupted. "We will need their experience to guide the new batch and overcome the difficulties and if the company feels they are productive in the times of recession, they can be retained after 6 months. Once the special managers are functioning it is the company's decision to keep or to fire the existing assistant managers" Tom replied

The CEO smiled and whispered in his ear, "**What a comeback!** I knew we had the right guy for the right job and wouldn't be long, one day, you will be seated in my chair".

<u>3.</u>

Frank

The default state of the mind is awareness i.e. is happiness....it's the inclination and dependence of the mind to save the information and relate it to the emotions generated gives rise to turbulence and noise in a human mind. The more we believe in what we feel rather than what it is, the more unhappiness we generate.

Sam was really excited to meet up with his friends after a long time. He was eager to meet his schoolmates, especially the ones who had taken immense pleasure in teasing and bullying him in school. He had always been a studious and frail boy who was a regular 'pick' for all the bullies in school. He was sure his friend Frank, against whom he had the maximum grudge, would be shocked to see him. Not that Tom was having any ill feelings towards Frank today, but he was eager to see Frank's facial expression, when he would see the transformation of Sam's attitude and behaviour. Sam had heard that Frank had been recently laid off from his company. His old childhood day's rivalry seemed to have given him that extra boost of confidence after hearing the news.
Sam's information about Frank was very much true and Frank was sitting unemployed and sulking at his house. Recently Frank had been into a lot of fights and had been to the police

station for assaulting a colleague in his office.
Things weren't so bad in Frank's life before.
Actually, Frank was from an affluent family and
was considered as one of the most flamboyant and
versatile speakers in school days. Since he was
the only child, he was pampered by his
grandparents and parents. From early days he had
the habit of getting whatever he wanted. He
would throw a tantrum if the family would not get
his wish fulfilled. His mother did try to correct
him many times but it would end up in a quarrel
with his father. Things were great for Frank until
he turned eight years but then his parents started
paying less attention to him. There would be
fights between his parents. Frank's father was a
chronic alcoholic and had an extramarital
affair. This would create a lot of arguments
between his parents. There would be squabbles on
small things in the house, like paying the
electricity or telephone bills. Altercations would
turn violent with Frank's father would beat his
mother at the smallest excuse. Frank's mom
didn't want him to see this, so she would send
him to her friend's house. Little Frank could see
the bruised face of his mother the next day but
would never ask her. He tried to confront his
father a couple of times. Once during such
confrontation, Frank's father threw him on the
table. Frank lost his balance and fell on his hand
and fractured it. This was the trigger point for his
mother. She decided to leave the house and file
for a divorce. Frank was ten at that time and it
was a very tender age. It was very difficult for his
mom to explain to him the meaning of divorce.
Actually, the reason behind Franks anguish was
that he was always very attached to his father and
considered him as his role model. The sudden

change in his behaviour was, because he believed
that his father was under a wicked spell by
another lady, and was not in his senses. This was
explained to him by his grandmother. Little Frank
never understood why the spell never came off.
Since Franks mother was a single parent after the
divorce, and she made his father pay her a huge
sum as a divorce settlement. Frank always got
what he demanded. When in school his friends
used to get 10 dollars a week, Frank would get
100 dollars. It was obvious for all the kids to like
him as he would throw a party every second day.
Everyone wanted to be his friend. So during his
school-time, he rarely had any altercations as all
the kids wanted to be with him. He would bully
and make fun of his friends who were a bit shy
like Sam. His grades were always poor, and he
would bully his friends into doing his homework
and his projects. He was a very good soccer
player and was selected for the inter-school team.
He was their star centre forward but in one of the
matches, the referee gave him a yellow card for a
foul. Frank felt the decision was biased and
wrong. He had an altercation with the referee, and
he hit him on his head. The referee was rushed to
the hospital, but no criminal charges were forced
against Frank, considering the age of the boy. His
mother never scolded him for the irresponsible
behaviour instead would blame the referee for his
wrong decisions. She was partially right because
that decision resulted in Frank's team losing the
game. He was banned by the inter-school
organisation for playing any further matches and
this greatly upset Frank. He agreed he shouldn't
have hit, but he blamed the referee for his bias
decision. This incident made Frank more
aggressive, and he would pick up fights with

people even for small disagreement. The school complained about his behaviour to his mother, who would pacify them, by telling them that he was undergoing treatment. He was referred to a psychologist for anger management where after the first two sessions he refused to go. Finally, Frank's mom changed his school and the problem was temporarily resolved. Frank had many heartbreaks when he was in college. He could never get involved in serious relationships. After some time he would start getting bored and would eventually find a reason to break up with the girl. However, times had changed, Frank's mom had just lost her job and there were financial crunches in the house. Frank had to take up a job. He would attend college in the daytime and would work in the night. In a span of three years, he had changed more than fifteen jobs. Some because of his behaviour, others because of his laziness. He would not show up without any prior notice. This would, of course, irritate his boss, and they would reprimand him. This would lead to an altercation, which would finally end up Frank being fired. This was a common story in most of his jobs. He finally completed graduation, but by that time, his house was in severe financial distress. They had to shift to a rented room and Frank started realising that he had to find a permanent job to support the house. He worked hard on improving his skills. He took classes for personality development and went to counsellors for anger management. His girlfriend Ivanna was very supportive of him. She would sit with him hours rehearsing how he should behave with his colleagues and his bosses. He applied for a job of a supervisor in a multinational company and finally, luck was on his side. He got the job with a good salary. He was also assured that he would be made permanent after seeing his performance for a whole year. Frank realised how badly he needed the job. He needed money to pay his loans and get married to Ivanna. Ivanna had a special place in Frank's life. Unlike his previous girlfriends who would come behind his money and luxury. Ivanna would listen to him for hours and would care about him. She was the only person, Frank felt who understood him, in this cruel world apart from his mother. They were deeply in love and were planning to get married, once Frank settles down.

It was his first day of job, and Frank wanted to make a great impression on his boss and colleagues. So he wore his favourite shirt, and reached office early. He had a decent first day, when Frank tried to be extra nice and courteous. The next week went on really well. Frank for the first time in his life felt that this was the right job he was looking for. Most of his office colleagues were very helpful and polite except Marc who had a temper issue. He was known for his arrogance and rough language. His habit of dominating people, and speaking roughly had caught people unaware. Still, everyone used to tolerate him because he was a distant relative of the Directors. He was given the job of a financial advisor in the company, but he would poke his nose in every department. There had been instances where people had been sacked because of Marc complaining to the director. So getting into an unnecessary conversation with Marc was a big no-no in the office and Frank was aware of it from day one. He would overlook his language and would try to be out of his way.

It was almost one month of Frank's new job, and

he was happy that he was comfortable with the new job. It was a Saturday, so he had decided to propose Ivanna for marriage while they were meeting for dinner on that day. He had to submit the project in the meeting, which he had been working since the last month. His manager was very impressed, with the gist of the project he had presented before him, a day before the final presentation. Frank was sure he would impress everyone with the presentation. He reached the conference table on time. The directors and manager were there. This was the chance Frank felt where, he could make an impression and probably get a promotion. He gazed around the room, and was delighted as Marc was missing. Frank knew Marc would not come to work on weekends, so he was sure that there would not be any interference in his presentations. Marc had given a tough time to many of his fellow mates in their presentation, just to impress the director and score brownie points. Frank knew he could not take this negative and sarcasm and had planned to make a presentation when he was absent.

Finally, it was Frank's turn to speak. He started the presentation with an impressive pictorial and graphical data. His audience seemed to be engaged with him, which made Frank feel very confident. Suddenly from the corner of the room, he saw a shadow entering the room. He tried to concentrate on the presentation, but the fear that Marc might turn up was distracting him. His worst fear came true. It was Marc who entered the room. He never turned up for work on a weekend, but he had come because he was planning to go for another meeting with one of the directors after this one. He was waiting for him in the lobby, but since he got bored, he decided to come up to the room. Marc was irritated as he did not like to wait for anybody. But this was one of the company's director, and he dare not rub him on the wrong end. He had heard a lot about Frank and his dedication to the work from his colleagues. He would come on time and would work till late evening, beyond company hours. "This lad seemed to be on a mission", one of his directors had once commented. Marc was a very insecure person and would get disturbed with even the smallest of things. In Frank, he had started seeing "a potential rival". He was waiting for an opportunity to pull him down. He saw him presenting a new concept which sounded really interesting. Everyone in the room seemed to be impressed with the concept. He decided to sit for some time and listen to the whole thing, before making any comment. Frank couldn't believe his luck and wished Marc would not engage with him in an unnecessary conversation. "Unnecessary conversation" was the word used in Frank's office for irrelevant and provocative questions, which were not related to the primary subject matter, which Marc loved to do. He was about to finish when Marc interrupted Frank and asked him, where had he copied this concept and idea from. He had heard this idea before and this had been tried in a company in France before. The company had to incur severe losses. Frank wondered how he came to know about the French project. He had not shared with anyone except his manager. Frank knew he could no longer avoid this guy. He answered, "There were a few points in his project similar to the one implemented in a company in France but. "Before he could complete Marc shot at him, "How dare he present a stolen idea from a company which had already made losses in the same project. How dare he come up with such ideas especially in an official meeting with the director and senior management? This showed his mental bankruptcy and lack of common sense". Frank tried to defend that he had added only a few points from that plan and rest was according to the present market scenario. Frank could feel the surge of anger growing in him with the rude remarks, Marc was making. Marc exploded "if you believe that people in this company are fools to listen to such bogus ideas, from dim-witted and thieves who steal other company's failed projects, than you are in the wrong place". He needs to get his head examined first". Before sanity could be established and someone could intervene, Frank whose was boiling like a volcano blurted out to Marc. "People who are feeding like parasites on companies expenses and are only surviving because of their proximity to a few senior people. They had no business to advise him". Suddenly Frank's old school bully behaviour comes to the forefront. "You are nothing but a burden on the company and if you didn't have the right relationship you are not even fit to clean the toilets in this company. You are nothing but a stinking garbage which everyone has to bear in the company". By now Marc had lost his control. Nobody dared had the guts to speak to him in this tone. He abused Frank and his upbringing for this behaviour. Frank by now was already on a point of no return. He picked up the showpiece next to him and threw it at Marc's head. He had a good aim and this hit Marc on his head blood started trickling down Marc's face and he fainted. Frank got scared. He couldn't believe what he had done. Luckily Marc was rushed to the hospital and was fine. He had a few stitches in the emergency room(ER) and was discharged. A police complaint was filed by the company and Frank was arrested. Frank couldn't believe he was behind bars and the things had turned around so fast. He strongly believed that this was the best way he could have responded and felt no remorse. The only fear was losing Ivanna which made him scared. He saw Ivanna talking to the officer. He felt relieved that Ivanna was there and when he met her, he told her, "That man deserved this. Wait till you hear the whole story". Ivanna had got a lawyer and arranged for a bail for him. Before Frank could explain anything else, Ivanna told Frank she needed some time to rethink about their relationship and whether she can deal with his behavioural problems. She left the police station and Frank who was already released on bail found his way from the police station to his house, long, difficult and lonely. He didn't know why Ivanna was angry at him or what was wrong in the way he had dealt with Marc who was talking rubbish. What was the need for him to work in a company where employees' are bullied? His self-respect was more important than anything else. At least he tried.

Insights

Frank right from his childhood was a pampered child, and he had never learned the lessons of inhibiting his thought process. His grades were poor because of his inability to suppress the urges. If he wanted something, he would have it. Being over pampered by his parents and guardians created issues of perseverance and arrogant behaviours in Frank's adult life. His habit of dominating others and bullying them also signifies the lack of empathy and the need to be accepted in the society. Bullying and ragging are a classic example of our need to be accepted in the society and being intolerant to others views. There is always a history of abuse in the family, where the child feels that it is the only way to put forward their views.

Bullying is existing in all schools and colleges but when it starts harming other children, it gets highlighted. The core problem here is the lack of empathy in parents who themselves are dealing with a lot of stress. There are very few educational institutes which teach children the lessons of empathy, right from kindergarten. Franks mind was continuously exposed to these situations and as he grew up, his cravings for the same recognition and satiety was not matched by his financial situation. He had to take lessons to be able to understand others and communicate without being too pushy or dominating.
Many people when they start working must have realised the lack of effective engagement skills and take these popular lessons in their adulthood. Emotional Intelligence and communication skill interventions have become highly popular because of the same reasons. However, Frank was forced into accepting these skills. He could not break free from the automation of his mind-set, created in his childhood, when he faced an uncomfortable situation. This created more unhappiness and sorrow. We may adjust to the changing situations but if the automation is not broken, we are not able to change our thinking process and get easily lured into our fixed mind-set. This is a tedious task for our brain which is more than happy to keep us in the fixed mind-set,

hence amplify our sufferings. One of the few examples where our mind resists changing our fixed mind-set is the ones who keep blaming others for their own faults. This is the best way one can fool themselves into believing, that fixed thinking about the given situation is the only way. Let me give you an example a fixed thought in our brain, say, "if someone pushes me I have to push him back without thinking about the consequences". If I don't, the other person might think I am weak or the other person provoked me, hence I pushed him. These are the common excuses our brain gives to defend its fixed thinking. Although it sounds very simple we keep making decisions on this rigid thought and increase both our anxiety and sufferings.

As for Frank he needs to spend more time with himself and rethink how to change his thought process. It may take time until he is convinced about his shortcomings.

We know that the mind stores information in the form of an image. When we register an image initially, we save it with the relevant emotions in the hippocampus. So when the similar incident is played out, the Hippocampal -Amygdala circuit gets activated and the same emotions are experienced. The mind tends to find similarities in the new experience it faces, and links it to the past incidents. Similarities as simple as colour, shape, similar language or preference makes the past circuit activated. Hence when we meet new strangers, we have that uncanny feeling of fondness or dislike, which seem to have no logical explanations. When the circuits get activated repeatedly, the pathways become stronger and stronger. Later on, the circuits do not need to wait for the whole experience, just the thought can activate the circuit and a person can experience the emotion. Like when we remember a vacation with our loved ones, where we had a lot of fun in the past we immediately experience happiness. If we meet an old school friend whom we had a lot of fights many years later, we experience the same negative emotions. The intensity does reduce if we experience it after a long time. But as we refire the same neuronal pathways, they become autonomous. Staying in a state where we have less control and are emotion driven, is not only the simpler and 'less effort option' for our brain, but it also gives rise to more unhappiness. Happiness is a mental or emotional state of well-being which can be defined by positive or pleasant emotions ranging from contentment to intense joy. The more the brain reacts to situations in an autonomous way the more the unhappiness.

Change is one phenomenon which is present everywhere. Hence the reactions to people, place, and situation have to also be appropriate. "Nothing remains static and has to undergo change" is a fact which we all have to live with. The human body, relationship, and even situations change as we grow up. But the automation we form in our neuronal paths tends to remain rigid. This creates misery, and the more we surrender to it, the more the brain pathways get rigid in this ever-changing world. Being autonomous, also means that there is no voluntary control over it. Repeated stimulation of these neuronal pathways creates permanent changes in the receptors and synapses. These facilitate stronger and faster stimulation of the brain pathways.

Coming to Frank, he did try to break the automation in his mind about being a bully and being impulsive and aggressive. He was forced into doing so because of the pressure from his degenerating financial situation and the love for his girlfriend Ivanna. Although he did put an effort trying to change his impulsive reactions and controlling the irrational behaviour, his autonomous neuronal paths were restimulated by the provocative words by Marc. These neuronal paths were dormant, not extinct, like a volcano waiting to erupt, they fired with full intensity resulting in losing his temper and physically assaulting Marc. The only way out is self-introspection of his behaviour and being aware of the malignant emotions, which created trouble for Frank in both personal and professional life. If he has to engineer a **comeback**, the only way possible is by, self-realization. Ivanna gave him the necessary space so he can learn from his mistakes.

4.

Hemant

Sam had spoken to Frank regarding his party and invited him to come, since he was planning to have a small get-to-gather of school friends in the party. They hadn't met for a real long time and it would be a great. Frank reluctantly did agree as he was going through a tough phase in his life. He didn't want to miss the opportunity and it would be a welcome change, after what he had gone through. He informed Sam about Hemant, an Indian boy who used to study in the class with them. He had recently met him in a restaurant and had interacted with him. In school, Sam used to gel with him a lot because of the many similarities in their behaviour. Hemant was also a very quiet and studious boy. He was one of the top rankers in the class and all of them would tell him that he would be a scientist one day. He was a perfect "rule following" child as we say 'a law-abiding citizen 'in adult life. Hemant was the teacher's favourite and would be the head monitor every year. He was afraid of Frank in his school-days because of his huge built. Frank used to bully him into doing his homework and steal his notes. Both Sam and Hemant came from middle-class families. Both were quiet from early childhood. Both were very good in their studies. However, Hemant came from a much stable family background. His family had shifted from India recently when Hemant joined the school. His father was a doctor and was a very busy man. He would rarely have time to spend with his son Hemant and his daughter Alisha. They used to spend most of their time with their mother Renuka.

Renuka was a software engineer and had stopped working only to give her complete time in raising up their children. It was mutually decided by the couple that Hemant's father would go to work and Renuka would manage the house. Renuka was always a dedicated and efficient employee, and would get praised by her seniors for her dedication. She would put her hundred percent in whatever task she was assigned. She always believed that discipline in life was the only way to achieve your goals and targets. You couldn't blame her for being so strict and disciplined because, this was the teaching given to her by her father who was in the navy who was very strict with her. Renuka was a loving but a very strict mother. She would not tolerate indiscipline especially if it was related to their academics. She would let the children play for fixed hours in a day, and at times would play with them as well. But when they would sit down for studies, she would not tolerate any hanky-panky. She would threaten the children with punishments, if they didn't listen to her. If she had planned to finish a particular lesson in the given time, she would not let the children sleep or eat. She would sit with them for the whole night until they completed their studies. Children at times would rebel against this military-like discipline, but Renuka would not budge. This installed fear and at times hatred for studies in the minds of children. In spite of her strict methods, the children would do very well in their academics. There were times when they would really miss their father, but he would rarely be available. The teacher never complained about their behaviour in school nor had issues with their academics. The children were disciplined and would do their studies on time. Only after finishing their studies that would go down to play. Renuka was a proud parent, and she felt that it's because of her discipline, that the children were doing so well in their academics. Renuka's influence and control of children started diminishing as the kids grew up. They started spending more time with their friends. Renuka used to feel insecure and scared that the children might spoil their future. Hemant particularly started rebelling and stopped listening to her. He would spend more time in the college library or loiter with friends. However, Alisha pursued her education and entered the medical stream. Both the kids believed that it was her mother's effort that they were able to focus and concentrate on their studies. Hemant loved teaching school children and wanted to be an educator. Renuka wanted him to be a doctor or an engineer. Although his mother Renuka opposed his decision, Hemant decided to move out of the house and pursue his dream of becoming a professor. Meanwhile, Alisha was still very much attached to her mother, and she went on to become a surgeon like her father. Whenever there was a family gathering, his mother would always taunt Hemant about how he had wasted her hard work just to become a professor. Hemant would feel offended, but would avoid getting into an argument.

Hemant fell in love with an Irish girl Branda. In spite of the opposition from his family, especially from his mother, Renuka, Hemant got married to her. Branda and Hemant soon had a baby boy after three years of marriage. Hemant was working in a public school as a math's teacher. He was very good at explaining the concepts and children used to enjoy learning with him. The children were also scared of him because he would get very angry if the assignments were not done on time. His punishments were often very controversial. They would range from humiliating the kid in front of others to sending them to detentions. He never had physically assaulted a child, though he would demoralise a child if they failed to comply with his instructions. Parents and PTA had often complained to the principal and the management about these punishments, but there was a shortage of good Mathematics teacher. The school carried on with Hemant in spite of his weird ways of teaching. Branda tried to convince him that being so strict with small kids would create aversion from studying, but he would turn a deaf ear. This would end up

resulting in quarrels in the house,
so Branda stopped telling him to correct his ways.
At time's children used to really get agitated with
his dictatorial style and complain to their parents,
but Hemant was unaffected. He was sure this was
the only way he could teach them and without
discipline in life, they will not be able to focus.
He argued with parents that the children need to
train their minds in their early age, and he was
simply helping them to do so. Since it was a
public school and there were no
alternatives, Hemant continued as a Mathematics
professor in school. Many parents even supported
his style of teaching, as they agreed with him.
Children get distracted quickly, hence there
should be some rules enforced.
Hemant was oblivious of the fact that many
children had stopped liking the subject, and at
times were studying it only because of his forced
military like teaching. Their grades were not
improving. He did not believe it was he who was
responsible, rather blamed the parents and the
Intelligence Quotient (I.Q) of the children.
It was the beginning of the year of the seventh
grade. Most of the kids had been with Hemant last
year and were aware of his style of teaching.
Recently a new student had joined the school. He
was from Italy and his name was Roberto.
Roberto had recently migrated from Italy with his
mother. Roberto's parents were divorced recently
and Roberto was staying with his mom. Roberto's
Mom was working with the bank and since she
was a single mom, Roberto would spend most of
the time with the maid. Roberto was an emotional

and sensitive child. It was difficult for the child to cope up with the couple's separation. He used to miss his father a lot, and now his mom, as she went for work. Roberto would be by her side when she used to come back from work.

Roberto was very good in canvas painting. He would sit for hours painting sketches which were unique for his age. He had won many laurels in painting in his previous school in Italy. He used to hate mathematics and logical reasoning. The previous school class teacher used to be very patient and take extra classes with Roberto for explaining the concepts. Roberto, in general, was a quiet boy, but when someone used to speak rudely to him he would start crying. It was unusual for a boy of 12 years to cry, at a drop of a hat, whenever someone shouted at him. Roberto's mother tried to explain to him to voice out his feelings and had consulted a child counsellor regarding this issue.

It was the first day of school and Hemant was the class teacher of the seventh grade. He entered the class to see Roberto. He realised he must be the new boy everyone was talking about in the staff room. The other teachers were admiring the paintings drawn by a new seventh-grade boy in school. Hemant felt that by painting on canvas, you don't earn money. To be successful you need to improve your logical reasoning and memory. Although art makes you feel good, it doesn't give you money, was his belief. Hemant started the class with an easy algebra problem and told Roberto to solve it. Roberto found it difficult as he had never learned it in the previous school. Hemant patiently tried to explain to him the problem and told him to wait after school, so he could teach him the new

concepts. Hemant realised Roberto was a fast learner. He understood the concepts and was able to solve the sums easily. Roberto tried his best to understand the lesson. He realised Hemant was better than the teacher in his previous school. The next day Hemant again picked up Roberto to solve another problem. Roberto got stuck again with the same mistake he had made

yesterday. Hemant warned him to be attentive or else he will make him stand out. He gave Roberto plenty of homework to solve. Since it was a long weekend he expected Roberto to solve all the problems. Roberto tried his best to finish the assignment he had been given. But Saturday was the day he used to sit with his passion. He started painting a beautiful picture of a boy solving a Mathematical problem and his teacher helping him. It was a creative portrait with numbers flying into the child's head with the teacher in portrait collecting the fallen number. By the end of the weekend, he showed the picture to his mom who was amazed at the child's creativity. His choice of colours and theme was unique. She advised him to gift the portrait to his professor. The next day as soon as Hemant came into the classroom Roberto gave him the portrait. Hemant was amazed at seeing the child's creativity. It didn't look like a 12-year-old child's painting. He thanked him and reminded him about his homework. Roberto had partially finished the assignment as he had spent most of the time doing the painting. Hemant's eyes were red on seeing, that the assignments were not completed. He flung the book on the floor and threw the painting in the dustbin. He told Roberto that the painting did not make up for his laziness. He told him that instead of wasting time on the painting, he would be happy if he had done his studies. This was simply too much for Roberto to handle. He burst out into tears. This made Hemant angrier. He told him to stop behaving like a looser and stand up for his mistakes. He told him to stay back for detention, and made him stand against the wall. Actually, Roberto had never been through this kind of punishments and teachers' behaviour. He was terrified. Hemant told him to repeat the homework. Roberto was too scared to talk to his mother about the teacher. He quietly finished his homework by dinner time and went to sleep. Roberto's mother thought he must be tired, so she didn't disturb him. The next day Roberto submitted the homework to Hemant who lashed out at him with rude words. All the problems were wrong. He insulted him by calling him dim-witted and having less IQ. The words had a negative impact on Roberto. He reduced his diet. He would sit quietly at home staring at the window. This went on for a week. His mom thought probably these were adjusting problems which will sought out in a few days' time. Again, that weekend, Hemant gave Roberto a lot of assignments to be completed. He warned him to concentrate while doing them and not to make any mistakes. Roberto didn't do any painting that weekend. He tried his best to solve the math's problem. With hands shaking he submitted the assignment to Hemant on Monday. Hemant saw the problems and started checking them immediately. He applauded Roberto as the first initial problems were correct. Roberto heaved a sigh of relief. Suddenly Hemant's facial expressions changed. He tore the pages Roberto had submitted. He shouted at him that after explaining him so many times still, he was repeating the same mistakes again and again. His brain was like a 6-year-old boy and had stop growing. Roberto was shocked and dejected. He felt terrible and felt the whole classroom spinning. He lost his consciousness and fell down. This scared Hemant. He immediately called the school nurse. The nurse examined him and found his blood pressure had fallen down. His mother was called and was told to take him home. Roberto was conscious by the time his mom reached the school. Roberto was quiet and didn't speak to anybody. His mother got worried, and she decided to take a couple of days offs from work to be with her son. Maybe he was finding it difficult to adjust to his new school. She took him for a short vacation. The moment Roberto's mom would speak about school, Roberto would start crying.

She cuddled him and explained to him that she will be always next to him whenever he wanted. He started telling her about how Hemant had flung his portrait and humiliated him in front of the class. Tears rolled down his face and his mother could see that her son was terrified at the name of the Mathematics teacher. She went to the school the next day to meet the principal. She threatened to call the cops if the management didn't take any action. She got his counsellor's certificate to prove that Roberto was terrified by the mathematics teacher and was in depression. This scared the principal. He immediately called Hemant and inquired about the matter. After a long discussion with Hemant, and after consulting with the management, he sent Hemant on a long leave. He apologised to his mother for Hemant's behaviour but Roberto's mother wanted Hemant to be out of the school. Meanwhile, Hemant didn't understand that he was only half an hour with the child every day. How can that lead him to depression? He was only trying to help Roberto to learn Math's, and he was improving with time, which was evident by the recent exam he had taken.

Insight

Hemant was raised by strict parents, who like most of us want our children to be disciplined and be excellent in their academics. And like in most cases of primary school children, all the strictness was actually working with Hemant's grades always being on the higher side.
But Hemant was a creative person. He was studying only because he was forced to. One of the schools of thought is that being too strict created a dislike for education... Hence, when he grew up he stopped listening to his mother and made a choice of becoming a teacher. Parents in

their love and at times their fear, end up being too dominating and do not give space to their kids.

Hemant was not too happy with his mother's way of teaching. He could not revolt because his grades were very good with Renuka's methods. When he stopped listening to her, his grades fell down. His mind-set was rewired and fixed, that this was the only way a child should be taught. This created an automation of his thought where he was not aware of the effects on the child he was teaching. It is ironical that Hemant was subjecting the child to the same agony what he went through, his lack of awareness of the emotions of the child whom he was teaching. He would immediately develop a fear that if he didn't teach them the way his mother taught them, they would suffer.

This is a very common problem that we do not realise what the other person is feeling when we are too stuck up with our efforts to help them. Instead of helping them, we end up harming them. The more we connect our experiences to the emotions we felt in the past, the probability of us reacting in the same way and going through the same agony, is the end result. We believe in these images, and we simply do not comprehend what the other person is
experiencing. Hemant although liked Roberto s creativity, but he was so stuck with the old image and their related emotions that he simply didn't understand the situation. This creates hatred in children when the educator is completely unaware of the mental state of the child.

Hemant dragged the matter to the stage where the child lost his consciousness. It is very common for people to drive the other person into this pitiable state, because of the old images formed in their brain. He needed to introspect and realise that the shortcomings of his mother's ways and the impact it had on his mind. This could be only possible if he shared his thoughts with a neutral person who could guide him without being bias or judgmental. He was lucky to have an understanding wife like Branda who could relieve him of his sufferings and be a great educator as he deserved to be.

It was very evident that the Hemant childhood experiences with his mother's strict ways of teaching, had made Hemant's thoughts very rigid and fixed. Let us try to understand the changes that took place in young Hemant's mind and how it affected his thinking. His mother's strict but insensitive ways of teaching made similar circuits in his mind by a process called "mirror neurons". Repeated stimulation of this circuit made his thoughts rigid. This was reinforced by the reward circuit as in the case of a habit or addiction. Praise for following her instructions and adhering to the toed instructions made the thought process rigid. The neurochemicals released in the reward circuit is dopamine. Repeated stimulation of dopamine by the circuits in the caudate accumbens of basal ganglia leads to up-regulation of dopamine receptors. This makes the receptors change structurally to fire earlier and facilitate the neurotransmitters by the

process known as facilitation. This process was strengthened by the improved results in the academics. Hence, the thought that strictness and discipline was the only way to improve learning got reinforced in Hemant's mind. The basal ganglia-amygdala circuit was fired, when there was depleted dopamine stimulation in the brain, leading to fear that the child was not learning lead to anger and humiliation of the child.
Also, Hemant had suppressed his emotions and creativity in early childhood leading to defective empathy and weaker pathways in the Right Dorsolateral prefrontal cortex circuits which is responsible for socio-emotional behaviours. Hemant could not understand the pain of the child and lacked appreciation in the child's ability to draw. Although he knew that Roberto was extraordinarily talented in painting, he was unable to comprehend it because of the rigidity of thoughts and the emotions attached to it. His wife Branda did try to make him realize his mistakes, but the effect of early changes and repeated stimulation due to his childhood experiences made it difficult for him to realise the defect in his way of thinking. He could not understand the child's emotions and was more engrossed in imparting his teaching by threatening, humiliating the child thereby increasing his stress levels. Though the intention may be right, the execution created more harm rather than benefitting the student as intended by Hemant.

Hemant was dejected and depressed by the school

management's decision. He simply failed to realise his mistakes and blamed the child's parent for pampering him too much. When he reached home and met his family, he didn't speak to anybody. He skipped his dinner because of the fear of the humiliation of telling his family that he was fired. This was too much for his male ego to handle. Branda realised there was something wrong. She called up his colleague who told her what had happened. She knew what the real issue was. What she feared and fought with Hemant a few days back had come true! She knew he was not in the state to understand, so she gave him time. For the next few days, Branda was always by his side. She didn't ask him any questions regarding workplace, rather they would go to places when they had spent time during their college days, reliving those beautiful moments. Hemant was always busy in school, so they rarely had time to spend together. And finally, when Hemant was comfortable, he opened up to Branda. He told her about the incident and how the school had reacted. Branda asked him, "What was he worried about?" The job or the child? Hemant told her it was the child what was bothering him more. Then she explained to him that for the last couple of days, she had waited for him to speak rather than forcing him to talk. She also explained how the experiences of learning during his childhood were interfering with his teaching. Although he was very good at imparting knowledge to the kids, his behaviour was creating an atmosphere of fear rather than trust. She even asked him, how he would have reacted, if a similar problem came up and their son had a nervous breakdown because of someone at school. He had suppressed his emotions in his childhood, and they were now creating the barriers. He was unable to think clearly. She told him to relieve the experience what he had in his younger days and tell her what he felt? Hemant although didn't agree with her, but he decided to do what she said. The next few days Hemant stayed indoors trying to understand what Branda said. Although he couldn't remember much, he knew he would be very scared and at times sad, whenever he would study. He also realised that the moment he heard the word study or its related word, he would get a sinking feeling. It seemed Branda was making sense. Hemant didn't speak much. He wrote down, whatever he felt in a diary.

He learned many things about himself which he had never thought about or gave it importance. He made images remembering what he used to feel when his mother stopped him from playing or sleeping. Tears rolled down his face. He realized the suffocation and helplessness he felt when he was a child due to the autocratic ways of his mother. Branda saw her husband sobbing in the room. She expected him to be upset, so she had decided to skip work for a few days till things settled down. Hemant's face said it all to Branda. The pain in his eyes mixed with the guilt of Roberto was obvious. Branda sat with him the entire night as Hemant for the first time spoke about what he felt in those days. How his mother had stopped his drawing and football, so he could

concentrate on his studies. He loved doing them
but was too scared to tell her.
The next morning Hemant went to school to get
Roberto's home address. He decided to visit him
in the night, so he can meet his mom. He had to
speak to Roberto if he wanted to come out of the
situation. He rang the doorbell. Roberto's Mom
opened the door and was shocked to
see Hemant at the door. She threatened him that
she will call the cops. Hemant asked her if he can
speak to her and her son for a minute. He needed
to talk to Roberto as he did not want him to carry
the same marks, which he had got in his early
childhood. He pleaded with her to allow him to
apologise. He didn't want them to take their
complaints back, but he wanted Roberto to realise
that education and studies aren't that bad, and he
should not develop a dislike because of a monster
teacher like him. Tears rolled down Hemant's
eyes. Roberto's Mom knew he was ashamed of
his behaviour, and he was the best person who
could heal Roberto's scars. She allowed him in
the house and Hemant spoke to Roberto. He
apologised for his behaviour and asked him for
forgiveness. He gave him the drawing he had
made yesterday and told him that he was a
horrible painter. Hemant told Roberto that he was
lucky to be blessed with the extraordinary talent
of painting. Unlike him who never got the
opportunity to improve his painting. Roberto very
innocently told him that he was ready to help him
provided he would do his homework on
time. Hemant began sobbing in front of Roberto
who put his hand around and told him in his ears

"sir, you are the best math's teacher I have ever met. Please come back to
school". Hemant realised that the boy was a gem and how wrong he was. He thanked his mom and left his place, relieved finally that the child was fine.

He decided to apply to other schools and started typing his resume. The phone bell rang. It was from the school and the principal wanted him to re-join the school. Hemant's happiness knew no bounds. He hugged Branda and thanked her for helping him to overcome his
sufferings. Hemant had taken special permissions from his mother to learn to draw from Roberto. Roberto stood first in the class in the Mathematics examination that year. " Oh! **What a comeback**! Hemant told Roberto. Hemant was the most liked professor in school after that incident and would be promoted to the post of Vice-principal. And huh… Hemant's painting was accepted and was to be published as the cover page for the school magazine…. **All thanks to his drawing teacher "Roberto".**

<u>5.</u>

George

Being positive is directly related to the extent of being aware of the moment.

Sam was thrilled to have invited his school friends who had not met him for years. As he went for his daily morning walk, he remembered his childhood friend, George who stayed just next door to his house. They were staying there for a brief period till he was around 13 years and then had shifted to Germany. He knew his aunt who stayed across the street. He thought if he could contact her maybe he can find out about George. He really wanted his party to have all the people whom he was close to or had some impact in the past to be present for the party. Luckily his aunt had the number and Sam came to know he was staying close by. As Sam called George's mobile. A sweet voice on the opposite end answered.

"This is Dr. George clinic. How may I help you?" Sam was surprised as his aunt didn't tell him that George had become a doctor. He had always been a smart child but he never liked science, when he was a kid. He told his assistant, "He was his childhood friend. His ex –neighbour Sam." The assistant was surprised at the introduction. She hesitantly told the doctor about Sam. George thought for a moment wondering who this Sam was. He told the assistant to take his number down and he will call later as he was busy. Sam was shocked and regretted calling him up. He thought maybe George had become egoistic like most doctors are. He went to his work feeling sad,

how people change and lose their innocence as they grow up. George was a gastro surgeon and was lined up for a difficult gastro-jejunal bypass surgery, when Sam called up. He forgot about Sam's call the whole day, and was busy until late at night. He reached home late night where his daughter and his wife Cathie had already gone off to sleep. While eating food, he suddenly recollected the call his assistant answered. He had taken the number from his assistant. He tried to remember who this ex-neighbour was. Suddenly it struck him. It must be that 9-year-old boy who used to play baseball with him. The one with whom he had once saved a puppy from drowning. A smile came on his face. This was the most exciting news he had heard for a long time. He removed the number from his pocket and dialled it. It was midnight. Sam and his wife were already fast asleep. George heard a soft male voice, "Hello. Who is this?" "Hey Sam", said George in excitement "Sorry I didn't recognise you when you called up in my clinic, and apologies for calling up so late in the night. How's my puppy doing"? 'Puppy' was the code word used by them to address each other after they had saved a puppy from drowning in the stream in their childhood. Sam was happy after hearing the word "puppy". It was his childhood friend, George who was on the other side. He was extremely happy to hear his voice. Both the friends spoke for an hour recollecting the old days. George was extremely happy to connect with Sam, and he assured of his presence at the party, Sam was hosting.
This was the most positive thing that had

happened in George's life, in the recent past. The last few days had been a rough patch for him. Although his wife Cathie was supportive of him, George knew he had to act fast before it was too late.

George had shifted to Germany when he was just 13 years with his parents. His life had been very difficult until he met Cathie. A year after shifting to Germany his father who ran a company of manufacturing shoes, had a major loss. Labour issues had shut down his business and he was declared bankrupt. His father could not take the humiliation and committed suicide. This had a very negative effect on George's psychology. His mother used to do errands and raised George with great difficulties. Her only aim was to make her son a doctor. Unlike his father who had never gone to school, his mother sent him to high school and finally to medical school, with great difficulties. George had seen, how his mother would give her share of food and feed George, so he can focus on his studies. George was a bright child. He worked hard to reach medical school. He was given a scholarship for his specialisation in Gastroenterology, which came as a great relief. By the time he completed his graduation, George's mother was diagnosed with terminal stomach cancer. George wanted to be by his mother's side but, his new job was both demanding, and he needed the money to pay back his loans. He would rush down after his duty hours and spend time with his mother. This was the first time he regretted taking up the medical profession.

He was saving people's lives in the hospital and working hard to remove pain from their lives. He felt extremely sad that he was unable to save his mother and give time to her. After all the hard work his mother had put for him in his childhood, he wanted to give her comfort and spend time with her. But he was unable to do so, as public hospitals were overcrowded, and he was not granted leave. One day when he was doing his night shift he got a call from his neighbours that his mother had passed away. George broke down in the hospital. He was performing an important surgery when he got the call. He gathered his emotions and completed the surgery. The surgery was successful but instead of meeting the relatives which are the norm. George ran home sobbing like a small child. He reached home and cried holding his mother's hand. The next few days George was quiet. He didn't speak much to anyone. Although he went back to his work in a couple of days, he did not communicate much. George was grieving as he felt his only support, his mother was no more. He was sitting in his office when someone knocked at the door. It was a beautiful girl in her twenties with an elderly gentleman who entered his chamber. He told her bluntly that he was not seeing any patients and called his assistant. His assistant told her no but the girl barged in. The girl told Gorge, her father was dying, and he was the only hope he had. All the doctors had given up on his father's ailment and hence she was desperate to meet him. This moved George as he had recently lost his mother, and he understood the pain of losing someone close. The girl introduced herself as Cathie and gave George, her father's reports. Cathie's father had Gallbladder cancer which was engulfing the aorta. The surgery could be fatal, and he could lose his life on the operation table. George explained this to Cathie but Cathie said she trusted him and was ready to take the risk, rather than letting her father die a slow death. Something in George's eyes made Cathie believe he would be able to pull off the surgery successfully. And Cathie's belief in George came true. George successfully removed the malignancy from the body. Cathie was extremely grateful to George and developed a fondness for him. Cathie and George connected well, post the surgery, and they would chat for hours together on the phone. They fell in love with each other and decided to get married. The very night when they were planning to go for a honeymoon, George got a call from a minister, whose son had met with an accident and needed emergency surgery. George had already boarded the flight. He asked Cathie, what to do, and she lovingly told him that he needs to be at the hospital. George rushed back to the hospital and saved the minster's son's life. It was a difficult surgery as the patient had already lost more than a litre of blood and the patient was VIP so all the OT staff was very tense. George had the nerves and the skills to negotiate and ligate the bleeding points in time to save the minister's son. George was applauded by everyone, but he was worried about his new bride. He rushed home to meet Cathie who was looking sad and staring outside the window. Cathie didn't show it but was extremely sad. It was obvious, anyone would be. But she hid her emotions from George, so he could focus on his surgery. She had called up the airlines but there were no flights to the Bahamas for the next 2 days. The ones which were available, were already jam-packed. When he saw his wife's sad face, he realised that this was the second time in his life he regretted being a doctor. The couple's honeymoon was delayed for a month, as something or other came up but, Cathie never complained or made any fuss. George was very strict with his patients and was always very clear about what he expected from the patients, and would give a detailed explanation of the disease they suffered. At times when there was no patient compliance, he would get irritated and would lose his temper. He was a perfectionist and would research and find out the diagnosis if he wasn't sure. His compassion and dedication were the key factors, which made him a very effective and prudent surgeon. He had diagnosed many rare diseases which most of his colleagues failed. His risk-taking ability, especially in high-risk patients, made him a daring but a level-headed surgeon. So in general, George was considered in his city, as a young and dynamic surgeon who had a miraculous cure for many untreatable diseases. George was running his clinic successfully for the last 10 years. His schedules were packed one month in advance. People from faraway regions approached him for difficult and risky taking operations.

One such patient Mr. Joseph and his 35-year

daughter had flown from the neighbouring city to find a remedy for a stage 4 anal melanoma (incurable cancer around the anus region). They were accompanied by their relatives who stayed in the same city as George. They got an appointment with George a week back and were in his clinic at the given time. But George was held up in an emergency. This made him late, by a good 2 hours. There was a huge crowd in the lobby of the clinic. Nancy, Joseph's daughter was unimpressed. She hated to wait for anyone, and expected people to be on time. Also, the crowd and the noise got her more irritated. But she had to meet George, as all the doctors had refused treatment for her father and her only hope was George. As soon as she entered George's room, she taunted him by saying, "Making people wait is a habit and some people simply do not understand what others have to go through". George was already tired because of the exhausting surgery, he had just done and didn't have the strength to engage with Nancy. He chose to overlook the comment and started discussing the case. He realised that Joseph was a 76-year-old man was suffering from incurable cancer which had spread into neighbouring organs. He didn't have a prognosis for more than one year. He was having problems with defecation and the spread of the tumour to neighbouring organs was creating severe pain in the region. The remedy was debulking or reducing the size of the tumour which would reduce his problems. This is termed as palliative treatment in medical language. But even this surgery was extremely dangerous as this tumour was engulfing major arteries and veins and the tumour was extremely vascular. The risk of surgery was extremely high and not operating seemed to be the right decision. He informed the relatives of his decision. With tears in her eyes, Nancy pleaded for him to operate. His life had become extremely painful and was on morphine tablets for pain. Even Joseph told George that it would be better if he died on the operation table rather than dying every day with his pain. George suddenly felt the same sinking feeling which he had experienced, when his mother was diagnosed with a malignancy. He saw Joseph face, which was filled with pain and anguish. He explained to the family, that there was 90 percent chance of death on the operation table and even within one-month, post-surgery death was possible due to embolism. He would be taking necessary precautions, but there was a high risk. He went on to add that he agreed to take the risk only, because of the patients and families insistence. So he will need a detailed informed consent, so that the family doesn't hold him responsible, if any untoward result comes during or after the surgery. The family agreed except Nancy's elder brother Fred who had not come to the clinic. The reason behind him not coming was that there was a property dispute between Fred and Nancy. There were a video and a written consent taken from the family members before the surgery. The surgery was scheduled on Monday morning. George had researched the books on similar surgeries done by other surgeons across the globe. He was ready for the challenge. Passionate about his work, he started the surgery meticulously removing the malignancy carefully manoeuvring the great vessels, while performing this high-risk surgery. He had decided to video graph the entire surgery to show it to the relatives in case if there was an issue.

George was able to debulk the tumour and remove almost 90 percent of the tumour without any major damage. The vitals were stable and George sighed a heave of relief after a 6 hours long surgery. The standby vascular surgeon congratulated George on successfully accomplishing this daunting feat. George called the relatives and gave them the good news. George showed the video and explained to them how he had removed the tumour. Nancy and their rest of the family were grateful to George for the successful surgery. A male voice from the background suddenly said, "Are you sure doctor that my father will be alright and will not die because of the surgery." George was shocked at this question from a person who was never there for all the consultation and was calling the patient, his father. Nancy explained that it was her brother and the family ignored his advice and comments. George saw Fred's face and could feel, he didn't trust the results of the operation. He explained that the most difficult part was over and now we have to wait and see how he recovers. Fred told George that this surgery was done without his consent, and he had refused to sign the consent form to the family. If something goes wrong, he will sue George as he had

operated without asking him. He will not let
George live peacefully. George was shocked by
this statement but before he could respond, Fred
had walked away. Nancy and the rest of the
family convinced George not to worry, as Fred
was an emotional person and the entire family
was with the doctor. Within the next few days'
Josephs health improved quickly. He was eating
food on the fifth day. His complaints had reduced
dramatically. George was very proud of his
achievement. He had decided to submit a paper
on this case in World Gastro Surgeons Meet. He
was sure he would be greatly appreciated for this
daredevil surgery. The relatives were extremely
grateful to George and his team and were praising
them for the wonderful care. On the eighth day
suddenly Joseph developed breathlessness and
was shifted to the ICU. George was on a vacation
as he hadn't taken a break for a really long time
and had told his colleague to follow up the case as
he was not in station. Joseph was recovering well,
so he was a little relaxed. A call was made from
the intensive care unit to George who
immediately realized that something had gone
wrong. His colleague told him there was no need
for him to come but George because of his
attachment and dedication for his work, decided
to fly back. He had an intuition, that it was not a
simple issue of breathlessness. He reached the
next morning to the hospital where the entire
family was standing outside the intensive care
unit. Fred gave him a stern look before he entered
the ICU. He spoke to his friend who informed that
Joseph had a suddenly developed a breathing

problem and before they could resuscitate, he had passed away. Probably it was due to a clot which had formed in the limb vessel and had blocked the artery supplying lungs, which cause this massive heart attack. This is termed as pulmonary embolism, which is a common complication in such major surgeries. George had warned the family about this complication before. George felt disappointed at seeing that all his hard work and effort had failed. He came out of the ICU to give the family the bad news. As soon as George told them that Joseph was no more, Fred came ahead and caught George's shirt collar and pushed him. He picked up the chair and threw at him. Nancy alleged that this was due to the hospital and Fred's mistake. How could he die, when he was recovering so well? The brother-sister duo started abusing George and finally, the security guards were called in, and they were arrested. George was in a state of shock and disbelief. He had never faced this kind of patient violence and hatred. He knew he had done nothing wrong, and there was no negligence. The hospital ordered a post-mortem which revealed that it was indeed a pulmonary embolism. George was sued for negligence by Nancy and Fred. He was supported by his colleagues and the judge ruled out any negligence on the part of the hospital or George. But this had a negative effect on George's psychology. He was unable to sleep for a few nights. He started blaming himself for making the wrong decision. He even blamed himself for his mothers and Cathie's father's death. He went to his psychiatrist friend who told him that he was suffering from a mild depression, and he needed to take a break. George had stopped seeing patients and had not done a single surgery for one month. His confidence was shattered, and he was unable to hold the knife which was once his strength and his belief. This was the third time in his life, he regretted being a doctor. He couldn't believe that people who considered him next to God, had suddenly turned him into a devil.

I can bet everyone agrees that being positive in life is the right attitude for being successful and resilient. But the most common question asked is why does our mind wander into negativity? Is there any scientific basis to this? GABA (gamma butyric amino acid) is the neurotransmitter responsible for inhibiting the impulse flow through the neurons and dopamine is the neurotransmitter responsible for the easing the flow of thoughts. Serotonin is another neurotransmitter which increases the receptors to bind with the dopamine neurotransmitter thereby increasing the impulse. The prefrontal cortex and the limbic system shows an increase in activity when our awareness is increased. The RES (reticular activating centre in the midbrain which plays a major role in keeping us alert. So when we get aware, the above circuits get activated. This is, in turn, gets more attention to the thought or impulse generated.

There is a natural bias of brain circuits and thoughts of negativity due to our genetic as well as experiences as we grow up. When we put our attention on a particular thought, we tend to generate more dopamine or positive thoughts. The prefrontal lobe through awareness of the given situation filters the negative thoughts. Although it sounds very easy, it is extremely complicated in a real-life scenario. There are many times in spite of awareness being present, the dominating thought will give enough alternative views justifying it. Since there are billions of neurons and trillions of connections. Awareness needs to be present for adequate time to make a tangible effect and come with an out of the box or a non-judgmental view or solution.

Let's say when we try to focus on a difficult problem or situation and want to find a solution. The most important criteria for a long-term and effective resolution is being non-judgmental and filtering, if not stopping dominant thoughts, so new ideas and thoughts are able to generate and new pathways can be created. All this requires a lot of awareness in the thought process. This is termed by many in today's world as "Out of the Box" thinking while others still call it lateral thinking. When the mind comes in full awareness of a particular thought, the negative thoughts or thoughts creating doubts seem to be less effective until and unless coupled with strong negative experience. The new idea thus created is more positive and effective. This goes a long way in creative and innovative decision-making which is a must in today's competitive world.

Insight

Dr. George had seen his parents sacrificing many things right from his birth, in spite of being in severe losses. This is common in most of the household. But in his case, he had seen them struggle more, since medical education requires a lot of money and his father was bankrupt. He was attached to his mother and wanted to be by his mother side when she was diagnosed with cancer. The profession he chose was demanding. The most common complaint of the doctor's family is that they do not give adequate time to them. This made him feel horrible especially when he wasn't beside his mom when she died. Dr. George blamed his profession rather than the situation.

So he felt that his profession was responsible, not the situation for his sufferings. Life is unpredictable. Most of the situations we face always have a surprise for us. Most of the things happening around us are not within our control except how we accept the situation.
The same thing happened when he got married and had to leave Claudie alone. He wanted to do medicine because his mother's dream. Hence it wasn't entirely his decision. He was brilliant and a very successful surgeon, but deep down in his mind, there was a fixed thought that he hated medicine. He was attaching the bad experiences, he faced in the medical profession.

The patient-doctor relationship is a relationship of trust and belief. Most in the medical profession have joined the field with an intention of empathy and compassion. But as years go by with the hardships, people change their behaviours but the intention never dies. This is one of the reasons why doctors have maximum job satisfaction.

He met a patient who was ungrateful which again is common in most of the professions. You may have a good customer who appreciates, and a bad customer who whines, no matter what you do for them. We meet people who appreciate our work and others criticize. The assault on him made him go back to the negative automation of thought, he had been harbouring for a long time. He wasn't thinking about the countless nice patients he had met but was stuck with one patient who had been so ungrateful. It was important for him to be aware of the compassion for him with which he served the patient.

 There is a negative bias in all of us partly because of inheritance and partly because of our experiences. Hence, Dr. George was stuck in the negativity and it needed his family or friend to help him overcome this fixed thinking. He needed to change the way he looked at the situation and not judge the profession on one bad experience.

Dr. George was unable to digest the rude behaviour of the patient who initially trusted him with their relative's life and then backtracked their statements. Although legally he may have been proven innocent, something inside him gave away. As per the advice of his psychiatric friend, Dr. George decided to go to his aunt's farmhouse. This was the perfect break Cathie was looking for. She was worried about her husband. George's aunt was a quiet place with animals grazing on the grass, rivers flowing nearby and a blue spruce tree in the backyard. George felt he would have been happier if he had been a farmer. People would have fewer expectations from him, and he could live his life peacefully. Cathie smiled at his sarcastic comments. She had got a list of successful operations, which George had done last year. She sat with him and asked him to recollect all the surgeries and how the relatives had thanked him.

One of the cases where he had operated on a single working mother, six months back. Her child-aged-8-years had made a wonderful card for him. Cathie had got the card to show it to George. Tears filled his eyes when he recollected how innocently the child had thanked him for saving his mother.

Then George suddenly interrupted, "why on earth the last surgery took such an awful turn?" He had done his best, and he had warned the family of the risk involved. Actually, he was not willing to operate but was forced by Nancy, the patient's daughter. It was unfair to him as a doctor to be slapped and thrashed by relatives when there was no fault of his. Cathie inquired, "Did George blame himself for the death." George sheepishly said "Yes and no". 'Yes' because he agreed to operate and 'No' because he had explained the risk to the relative".

Although, he was a professional he did not get emotionally involved with patients but at times the aggression to cure the patients gets him obsessed with the outcome. Cathie added, "That is normal and everyone in their profession does get passionate about their work". This gave George the drive to take on difficult surgeries and the expectations rose with initial success. She asked him once again, when the relative slapped him what did he feel? George innocently replied "he felt unhappy because they chose to ignore his efforts". He was angry because he chose not to listen to his inner voice that said not to 'operate'. He felt his hard work was not appreciated. Although he did understand the loss for the family was great, and they were reacting under stress.

She asked him again," why did he lose his confidence in the profession". George replied this profession had given him a lot of sorrow. First his mother, then their honeymoon and finally he got beaten up because of it. He had joined the profession because he wanted to relieve people of their problems, not to get beaten up. Cathie asked him to remember the times when he was proud of himself for being a doctor. There were plenty of such instances and Georges face suddenly lit up. He realized that he has helped people in their most difficult times. He was lucky to be able to make a change in people's lives. Still, he was not convinced whether he wanted to start operating again.

Suddenly a boy and his mother came in the car and waved at him. It was the same lady Cathie was talking about. She had a lump in her small

intestine which was operated by George. It was the same boy, who had made him a card and thanked him for saving his mother's life. The boy ran to George and hugged him. He told him to bend as he wanted to share a secret. The boy whispered in George's ears, "I met a fairy godmother yesterday in my dreams. She told me that she had been busy and couldn't go around everywhere. So he sent her assistant to help people around. Mom told me you were upset" the boy said. George smiled at Cathie and asked the boy, "Can I meet that assistant as I need him badly. "The boy removed a plastic toy from his bag. "Here, he is! "The boy exclaimed. He showed George a mirror on the backside of the toy. "The fairy God mother told me that you are one of her assistants. But who will solve your problem. I am small, not a doctor like you". George became very emotional at the innocent words of the child.
He looked at him and told him you are the angel who will help me and hugged him.

The boy innocently told him, "Don't stop going to hospital. There are many boys like me whose mother are not well. They need you."

This meeting was planned by Cathie to cheer George up, but she never expected the little boy to tell his dreams to him. George thanked them for coming and visiting him. He told Cathie to give him his mobile phone. He wanted to call the hospital and plan for the next surgery. Cathie looked at George lovingly and told him that she

would have to once again wait for him to come
home late.

6.

Thomas the businessman

Competitive neuroplasticity is a phenomenon taking place every moment of our life and is highly underrated by our experiences.

Sam was very excited about making the party a grand success. He wanted to give back his old times, connect with old friends and try to pull the hands of the clock back to those old and beautiful moments which he cherished. He was very clear he wanted to call everyone from his school and college life, who had contributed to his understanding of relationship in the present life. He remembered his college mate Thomas, who later went on to be a big businessman. He had spoken to him and his wife Zarine a day before and had invited him for the party.
Thomas from his early life was never interested in studying. He had struggled with his academics and was usually considered the dullest amongst the three siblings in his house. His elder brothers were extremely smart and very good in their studies. Thomas found it difficult to focus. He was a dreamer, and always dreamt of being a traveller. He loved to see new places and meet new people. At times, when his father used to send him for an errand, he would speak for hours with strangers.
Apart from his family, most of the people around

would share their problems with him and Thomas would patiently listen to them and help them with their problems. One of his neighbours had some problem with his cat's health. She was unable to visit the vet as she was too bedridden. Thomas took the cat to the vet on the day before his annual examinations. The result was obvious, he failed his exams. That was the day when Thomas's father made a decision, and he stopped telling him to study. He gave up on Thomas and his ways. He was already worried about his other two son's future, and he told Thomas he will never force him to study henceforth. Thomas tried his best to focus and concentrate on studying, but he simply could not get through his exams. After repeating every class twice he finally gave up on his education. Meanwhile, his brothers had become successful engineers and both were placed in multinational companies. As for Thomas he had barely made through the high school. He used to loiter the whole day with his friends and do errands for people. His father saw his son's irresponsible behaviours and finally decided to give him an ultimatum. He told him like his brothers, he has to pay for his stay and food otherwise he can leave the house. Thomas didn't believe what his father said, and he took his words lightly.

After a couple of days when his father realized that there was still no change in his behaviours, he decided to take things in his hand. One morning when Thomas got up, he saw his luggage was all tied up. He was shocked to see that. His father told him that he can leave the house and come back only when he has a job and can support himself. Thomas couldn't believe what he heard. He stormed out of the house angry and hurt by his father's decision. He went to his friend's house who refused to allow him to stay in his house. That night was the most difficult night of his life. He had to sleep under the stars without food in his stomach. He couldn't believe his fate. His friend and neighbours whom he had helped all their life had suddenly turned their back on him. He couldn't accept that he was so helpless. He vowed, that he would never go back to his house and one day become a successful person.

This was a life-changing experience for him. He decided to board a train for the city where he believed there were more opportunities. Without a single dime in his pocket, he travelled ticket less. On seeing the ticket collector, he jumped out of the moving train into the field. Thomas was a fighter, and he knew he had to survive this difficult time. He knew he was capable of turning the tables of fate and destiny. He realized that the world is a cruel place and his belief that empathy and compassion were the two most important thing in a person's life seem to have taken a bigger hit. His only aim in life was to earn more money than his brothers and to prove to his father and family that he was not "useless" as they had coined a word for him. Even after falling from the train his knees bruised and bleeding, Thomas got up and started walking toward the city. He followed the track and reached the city which was about 30 kilometres. Hungry and tired, he reached a food stall. He had no money in his pocket, and

he was hungry. The only way he could survive
was to steal.

By now Thomas had learned that he needs to
survive, no matter what he has to do. He planned
to steal a loaf of bread from the store without
being caught. He was successful in diverting the
attention of the shopkeeper and steal the loaf. He
sat alone in the deserted street eating the loaf with
tears in his eyes. He couldn't believe he had
stolen something. Although Thomas did not like
the school he was never involved in any criminal
activities. He went back to the store the next day
and met the shopkeeper. He told him that he had
stolen the loaf a day before and when he would be
a big man he will repay ten times the amount he
owed him. The shopkeeper was angry but also
amazed at the boy's honesty and confidence. He
decided not to punish him and simply told him
that he will wait for the day, when Thomas's
words would come true.

Thomas went to the city doing small jobs like
lifting weights or cleaning cars and started his
journey what he called "the survival of the
fittest". Darwin's theory and its application was
the only thing which he loved to read when he
was in school. One fine day while he was working
at a construction site he noticed that there was a
flaw in the building design. He went up to the
chief architect and pointed out the defect in
engineering. To this, the architect and the
engineer laughed out loud and told him to mind
his own business. The investor was a passive
spectator who heard the entire conversation. He
overlooked this incident as an over smart

employee. Thomas right from birth was a very keen observer and was the first one to pick up minor and subtle changes around him. He had no formal education on construction but his observation while working at various construction sites made him feel that there was something wrong in the design.

And it so happened a week later, part of the building collapsed leaving the chief architect and engineer in a dilemma. The investor came to the sight to see the damage and was grateful that there was no injury to anyone. He saw Thomas standing behind the crowd. He called him ahead and asked him how he was able to pick up the flaws. Thomas told him that he realized that the angle of the pillars was indeed not aligned as they should have been. The investor sought the clarification from his experts who concluded that Thomas was right and there indeed was a fault in the construction of the pillars. The investor was impressed and he lauded Thomas. He offered him to join his advisory panel and work as an assistant manager and supervise all his construction sites. Slowly Thomas because of his honesty and his dedication rose to the post of Chief Manager of all the sites. He learned all the tricks of the trade and in five years, most of the decisions in the company were always referred to him for the final opinion.

The first thing he did was to repay the loan of the shopkeeper whose bread he had stolen. He got married to his co-worker and his supervisor Zarine. Zarine was a very understanding and a patient lady. She had studied her majors in nursing and patient care but was working with the construction company as she was short of money and had her elderly parents to take care. She found, Thomas a very understanding and a loving life partner. Thomas became a very popular person in the company because of his friendly and understanding attitude. He had many friends but there were many old employees who became envious of him. But somehow he managed to work with them and extract work from them. Things looked very smooth for Thomas until the New Year's Eve. Thomas was returning home from work and was planning to go home. He started his car and drove on the busy highway to reach home. Since it was the eve of the New Year, there were many people who were drunk were walking recklessly on the street. So Thomas was careful in driving safely through the unruly crowd. Suddenly a young man with his group appeared out of nowhere. Thomas applied brakes but was unable to stop the car completely. The car went and touched the boy's knees. He had a mild bruise but his friend who was accompanying him got angry. They had been drinking since morning. They confronted Thomas and without giving him a chance to explain, they started thrashing him. One of the boys got an iron rod which was lying in the boot space and hit it on Thomas's head. Thomas lost his consciousness and fell down. The boys were scared but before they could escape the cops arrested them. Thomas meanwhile was taken to the hospital where he was diagnosed with a head injury. He had to undergo an urgent surgery in the form of

an evacuation of a massive clot from
his subdural region (space between the skull and
the brain). Luckily for Thomas, his life was saved
but because of the injury to the frontal lobe, he
could not control his emotions. He would burst
out in tears for trivial reasons or a sudden outburst
of anger for irrelevant issues. At times, he knew
he was overreacting, but he felt helpless. He also
was unable to use his left limbs. Although there
was a gradual improvement in the functions of his
left limbs, Thomas always felt his left limbs were
weak. He would limp and walk and avoided using
the left hand.

Zarine who understood his condition would assist
him in his chores patiently. She would motivate
Thomas to work more on his limb but it was
becoming an uphill task for him. At times his
sudden anger would upset Zarine, but she
understood his plight. It was four months since
the incident, but Thomas could not believe that
his life had changed. He realized that life would
not be the same again. He wanted the boys who
had hit him to get the maximum punishment. He
regularly met his lawyers to see to it that they get
the maximum punishment. He blamed them for
his miserable state. Although the boys and their
family had apologized to Thomas and paid all his
medical bills, Thomas could not forgive them. On
the contrary, he wanted to teach them a lesson. He
was determined to go after them until justice was
served.

Zarine tried to persuade Thomas that rather than
wasting time on the lawyer he should find ways to
improve his conditions and move on. This would

agitate Thomas, and he would speak rudely
to Zarine. He had already broken the television
set a couple of times in a fit of rage. The
management allowed Thomas to come to the
office in a wheelchair after 6 months as there was
a lot of a backlog. The change in his personality
was extremely difficult for his colleagues to
handle. He would be extremely impulsive and
would insult his colleagues for trivial issues. The
management found it extremely difficult to retain
him as Thomas was spoiling the work culture
which was actually was built by him. There were
many complaints registered against him in a span
of 2 weeks when he stayed in the office. Finally,
the company decided to suspend him indefinitely
and gave him the notice to mend his ways or seek
voluntary retirement. From an asset, Thomas had
become a liability to the company.
People stopped talking to him and whatever
conversations he had would create unnecessary
arguments. Thomas had been in difficult
situations before but there was always his
calmness and awareness which was his strength.
The absence of calmness and being over
impulsive, made it difficult for Thomas. Thomas
was extremely depressed for the next
week. Zarine decided to take him to the
psychiatrist but Thomas refused to take any
medications. This actually created more rifts
between Zarine and him. Once for a trivial
argument in a fit of rage, he hit her with the glass
showpiece. Blood was pouring from the cut on
her face. Thomas could not believe what he had
done. Zarine was rushed to the ER (emergency

room) and first aid in the form of suturing and medicines was administered. Luckily there was no internal injury. Zarine's parents decided to take their daughter away from the house until Thomas starts taking medicines or controls his behaviour. They warned Thomas to be away from Zarine. Thomas was devastated. He decided to end his life. With a blade in his hand, he wanted to put an end to his miseries. He couldn't believe, that the accident had turned him into a monster, who had started eating his family and friends.

We all have been trained right from birth to deal with competition. Forget after birth, there was a competition before birth, where one sperm won the race and fertilized the ovum and because of which we are existing in the world and reading my book today. Have you ever realized that we are existing today because the rest of the 1.2 million sperms lost and perished?
Well going forward, there is a competition everywhere existing around us. The two parts of any competition are that one is a winner and the other is a loser. Similar to this there is also a competition in our mind where one neural circuit competes with the other circuit. The one which is more aggressive wins the battle and that forms our decision and finally leading to a response.

So what happens to the other circuit is the burning question which is present in everyone's mind. Say for instance when we are very positive about a particular event, we get happy and chirpy and it reflects in our response. The circuits which are responsible for the negative view gets suppressed, and we are actually not aware of the negative thoughts we had in our mind. This phenomenon is called the competitive neuronal circuit. Let's go more into detail about how this affects the neuroplasticity in an individual. As we have discussed neuroplasticity is the ability of the brain to form new neurons and neural circuits. This is especially in case of anatomical recovery of any brain injury due to trauma or disease. This has been the reasons behind some miraculous recovery by stroke patients. New cells are generated, they rewire and are able to perform the functions.

This was observed by Bach-Y-Rita a neuroscientist where his father recovered completely in spite of a major part of his brain is damaged. In 1984, a team led by Michael Merzenich, a neuroscientist at the University of California at San Francisco, conducted experiments that began to explain phantom limbs as a true physiological response. Merzenich and his colleagues first amputated the middle fingers from a group of adult owl monkeys and later stimulated the digits on the hand of each monkey that was adjacent to the amputation stump. Placing microelectrodes, which detect electrochemical changes in actively firing neurons, into various areas of the monkeys' brains, Merzenich found that the region of the cortex that originally fired in response to stimulation of the amputated finger was now triggered every time he touched the two adjacent fingers. The neurons had not responded to stimulation of these fingers before the amputation.

In 1991, Timothy Pons, a neuroscientist at the Laboratory of Neuropsychology at the National Institute of Mental Health, expanded on Merzenich's findings. Working with adult macaque monkeys, Pons and his colleagues "deafferentated," or cut, nerves that communicated sensory information between the cortex and the arm, forearm, hand, and rear of the head. The team then stimulated various body parts and found that the part of the cortex that had previously responded to the arm and back of the head now responded to stimulation of the face. Like ivy spreading over bare brick, Pons believed that surrounding neurons invaded the fallow cortical area corresponding to the deafferented limbs, allowing it to respond to stimulation from other parts of the body.

Another interesting fact about the deafferentated monkey was that when they were left on their own the limb which was deafferentated did not move at all. But when the normal limb was plastered and not allowed to move, the deafferented limb was forced to come into action, it slowly recovered its complete function. This phenomenon is termed as competitive neuroplasticity.

When Michelangelo painted the Sistine Chapel, he had to work in an awkward position with his head thrown back looking up. During the project, his brain adapted so that he saw the world in that weird upside down way all the time. Upon completion, his vision took several months to go back to normal.

Studies have revealed that musicians, who play stringed instruments, have larger areas of their brains dedicated to their active hands. Brain scans of London taxi drivers have shown that the more years a driver has on the job correlates to a larger portion of their brain handling the storage of spatial relationships. Mediators exhibited denser parts of their brains activated when paying close attention to something.

So coming back to Thomas and his worries. Thomas from his early childhood had faced many difficulties, this by default had made him tough and resilient. In spite of being in tough situations, he had always been calm and composed. He had always worked for the solution rather than getting entangled in the loop of warring emotions. This had given him the ability to fight back and crawl out of problems. But now since his prefrontal lobe (regulator) seem to be injured and there was unregulated functioning of the amygdala causing him to be impulsive and highly emotional. Secondly, his left limb was weak, and he was suffering from unilateral paresis. This had an effect on his belief and state of mind which had shaken his belief and confidence. It is usual with post-traumatic stroke patients to have depressive episodes and so what Thomas was going through was pretty much the usual. The two strengths about his personality his calmness and his confidence seemed to be lost in the backyard of neuronal circuits which was creating all the troubles for him. The only way he could recover was that the brain areas which were not damaged start controlling his impulsive behaviours. Was it possible?

Insight

How the 6th law helped Thomas
Competitive neuroplasticity is a phenomenon taking place every moment of our life and is highly underrated by our experiences.
Thomas right from his early childhood was a people person. He loved to help people and was always ready to sacrifice many things for strangers. This is a perfect case of a right to left hemisphere working in coordination with each other. People with good communication engagement skills have good cross-hemispheric connections. This a quality which many people in their adult life crave for which Thomas was blessed from his early days. He was also a fighter and an optimist person who had fought many odds and build his stature in the company. His strength was his awareness levels which made him rise steeply in spite of not being educated. It has been observed that intelligence and emotional rarely walk together in an individual and those who have both have attained great heights. Even if we end up excelling in something, we become deficient in other things. It is humanly impossible to have all the skills in a single person. Hence, the role of teamwork and engagement becomes highly important in today's world.
The prefrontal lobe which has all the control over the emotional brain was damaged by the accident. Thomas had lost all his skills of controlling his emotion and alertness levels. This was

compounded by his physical weakness, which had a negative effect on his mind. He wasn't aware of the commotion in his brain and the changes because of the accident. This led to a series of events which he ended up harming his family and friends. The beauty of competitive neuroplasticity is that, one can make use of the parts which are not damaged, and compensate with it, if there are adequate inclination and motivation. Every negative event has a positive aspect provided we are able to see through. Thomas had many such positive reasons to look at, because of his inherent awareness skills. Being aware of the sudden change in the behaviour after an incident, it is difficult for many to comprehend. But that is the way forward where we can use the property of our neurons to overcome our shortcomings.

Thomas was sitting in the chair with a blade in his hand. He realized that he was a big burden to his family. He was extremely guilty and ashamed because of his erratic behaviour to Zarine and also felt helpless he couldn't do anything about it. He was sure that there was no point in living anymore as he would be harming his family and friends and it was better he ended this miserable life. Thomas picked up the knife and was about to make the first cut on his radial artery when he heard a sparrow chirping. He turned back to see where the sound was coming. Actually, when Thomas was young he used to spend a lot of time in the farm seeing the sparrow built the nest. He would see them picking up twigs and making a nest. He always felt inspired at seeing them rebuilding the nest even if the twigs fell off. The sparrow would again go in search of new twigs. Seeing them hunt for insects or grains and feeding their babies. He would feel happy whenever he was in some trouble, he would simply observe them running around gathering the twigs. Thomas went in the window to see if there was any nest nearby. And Voila! It was there, just opposite his building. A sheepish boyish smile came on Thomas' face. He experienced the same happiness which seemed to have disappeared since last few years.

Oh! My god! Thomas couldn't believe he had given up, and so he decided to postpone the suicide for a week and try to find a resolution. He always could do the same anytime next week, was the argument he made to himself. He sat down removed his diary and started making a list of his problems and their priorities. On the next page, he wrote down the probable resolutions. He realized the first thing he needs to do is to get his house in order. So he went to his wife Zarine's house. He met her parents, and he assured them that he would try to control his anger and would take any form of treatment. It would not be possible for him to recover without Zarine by his side. Tears rolled down his face as he spoke to her parents. Zarine who was secretly listening to the conversation ran into the living room and hugged him. She could see the guilt in Thomas's eyes, and she told her parents Thomas needs her, and she will help him to recover. Although her family didn't agree, Zarine was firm.

Next, for his anger, Thomas went for anger

management classes and hired a mindfulness coach to calm himself down. He wanted to get back his calmness which was both his necessity and his strength. He slowly started improving and was able to control his impulsivity and outburst. He decided to visit his office. He met his colleagues and apologized to them for his irrational behaviour. He sought permission from the management as he needed more time to get his act together. The management agreed to give him more time.

The next thing Thomas realized that he was not using his weak hand much. So he decided to do most of his work with the weak left hand and even tried to walk with Zarine's support with his left leg. He fell down a couple of times but this did not discourage him from getting up again. When he sat on the dinner table like a small baby would spill his food on his clothes. He would take hours just to write alphabets like a small child learning how to write. It took him 3 months to make a proper circle. This did not wear him down. He was determined to come back. Slowly his motor functions started improving. It took him a year to gain back his strengths. Once he was able to manage his emotional outburst and impulsive behaviour, he re-joined his office. Slowly he was back to handling difficult situations in the workplace. As he was walking back from work one day, he heard a sparrow chirping. A big smile came on his face as he turned back and thanked the sparrow for giving back his life to him.

<u>7.</u>

Lucy

The more the mind believes in the images it forms and the related past and its emotions the more the sufferings. The lesser it believes in the images it forms the more the scope for awareness and resolving difficult situations.

Sam was going to his office where he saw his high school friend Lucy. She had come with her husband and son for shopping. He invited her to the party which was scheduled for a couple of weeks. She agreed to come with her family. Sam couldn't help noticing the change in Lucy's behaviour. She was that typical tomboy types, outspoken and impulsive. She often used to have fights with boys both verbal and at times physical. Most of the boys were scared of talking to her. It was hard to believe Lucy speaking softly and calmly to Sam.
He asked her," What was the reason behind her transformation from a tough lady hulk to a polite lady". Lucy smiled at him and told him it was a long story, and she will tell him some other day. Sam told her that she would be one of the most popular people at the party because of her drastic transformation. Both laughed out loud. As Lucy walked ahead happily to meet her old mate, she thanked her stars, she was able to overcome her biggest obstacle in the recent past and was in the right state of mind to meet her old friends. As she

and her husband Larry were walking in the store, Lucy recalled how her childhood had such a big influence in her present life.

Lucy was born to a lower middle-class family. She was an unwanted child as both her parents were not expecting her. They both were just 20 years when she was born. Her father was yet to complete his college and her mother was a dropout. Her father James was a basketball player and hailed from a conservative family. The couple did not abort the child. Lucy mother was suffering from a congenital heart disease and in spite of the doctors warning, she continued with the pregnancy. Actually, the decision of the couple to keep the child was due to the insistence of James and his conservative views on abortion.

As expected by the doctor Lucy was born as a premature child but her mother could not survive the stress of the pregnancy. James was not very happy as he wanted a boy child. He didn't see the child's face for a good three-day post her birth, and she was left at the mercy of James's mother. Until Lucy was 10 years she was reared by James's mother. She always wanted to be around her father as he was the only surviving parent. She would behave and wear clothes like boys to make James happy. She would play basketball simply because James loved playing basketball and would appreciate her. Her hair was always short, and she would speak only to boys in school. The rest of the girl would tease her and call her "lady hulk". Lucy would often have brawls with her male friends, and she would beat them up black and blue. As she grew up she had more issues with interacting with boys. She could never trust any boys as she believed that boys always look down on girls and dominate them. She never had any girlfriends because there were no common topics which she could engage with them. She tried her hand with bodybuilding when she was in her high school and would work out for 6 to 7 hours. When she grew up, her father tried to make her understand to tone down her behaviour but it was too late. Lucy had endless bloody fights with the boys while playing basketball. Although she had a few casual affairs the relationships were short-lived because of her mistrust in a close relationship. She studied further and went on to become a sports trainer. She was a very strict person always forcing her students to be punctual and dedicated. She was highly appreciated because of her dedication and conscientious attitude. She still was very much attached to her father and would take care of him. He was the only relationship whom she blindly trusted and looked up to. James himself was an aggressive person and all his impatience and ruthlessness seemed to have passed on to his daughter. James met with an accident and broke both his femur (the thigh bone). He had to undergo an urgent surgical intervention and was unable to walk. He was bedridden for one whole year and need twenty-four hours of support and care. Lucy tried to help him for a couple of days but later she realized it was too much trouble for her and James was not making an effort and getting dependent on her. She kept a helper for him who would be with him throughout the day.

She expected James to deal with his everyday problems rather than calling her up. She would get annoyed if James would call up during her work hours or when she was in the club. Since Lucy was a trainer she had made a couple of friends with whom she used to party late nights. James's helper would leave by 10 in the night hence he had a lot of trouble with his everyday chores in the night. He could not even go up to the washroom on his own. He would call up Lucy again and again. Initially, she would answer his call but later she stopped picking up the phone. If she did come home early, she would simply tell him to manage it till morning. This would create a lot of fights between James and Lucy. Lucy simply could not understand why James was making a fuss about her night outs. She took it as one of his ways to bully her, which most of the males often do. This would create heated conversations. She finally decided to leave the house. James who had not completely recovered pleaded her not to go. But Lucy realized that if she would stay back James would be dependent on her and would never make an effort to overcome his disability. As Lucy left the house James realized his mistakes and what damage he had done to her psychology and her understanding of the relationship.

Her lack of compassion and empathy made him recollect the way he had behaved with her in her childhood. Whenever she was in fever he would force her to get up and do her dishes. When she had a fight with her friends, he would tell her to open the first aid kit and bandage her wounds on her own. He remembered when her first boyfriend left her and Lucy came home crying with her broken heart, James had told her to move on. He had told her that emotions were for weak people and the ones who cry send an invitation to the others to come and exploit them. As James remembered the past incidents, he realized what a horrible father he had been. He also recollected the number of times James had cursed Lucy's dead mother for leaving behind this burden on him. All this made James very unhappy. The next few days James did not eat much. He tried to call up Lucy a number of times, but she did not answer him.

One day when he was getting up from the bed, the floor mat came under his leg, and he tripped and hit his head on the glass table. He lost his consciousness for four hours and there was no one to attend to him. The helper came after four hours to his house where he saw James lying on the floor in a pool of blood. He called the ambulance and was rushed to the hospital. He had suffered a massive brain haemorrhage and had to undergo an emergency subdural evacuation. Lucy was called in by the hospital where the doctors informed Lucy that his health was critical. He would not be able to survive till the next morning. With tears in her eyes, Lucy went to meet James who was lying on the bed. She wanted to apologize for not being there when he fell down. James opened his eyes slowly and whispered in Lucy's ears. She does not need to feel guilty. She tried to do what she could. He was responsible for her behaviour, and he told her to promise him something. This was his last wish, but he wanted Lucy to promise him. Lucy although hesitant agreed as she was already feeling guilty about not being there. "Whenever your life is difficult and you are feeling helpless and there are no solutions you can see…always remember that everything in the world comes back if you cultivate compassion and empathy for people." James asked her to promise him that she would try to cultivate compassion and empathy in her times of crisis. This sounded funny to Lucy, but she had no choice but to agree with him. She did not want another guilt back on her shoulder. The next morning, James breathed last. Lucy lost the only person whom she trusted the most in the world. She knew life will change after her father's death.

Although Lucy had been showing a tough behaviour to her father, she was very much attached and emotionally dependent on him. She knew she will have a tough time to live without him. She continued her work and would spend more time in training to distract her mind from thinking about James. She met Larry who had recently started training in the gym. He was a software engineer and was working in a multinational company. Recently he was diagnosed with an abnormal lipid profile, so he was advised by the doctor to start exercising. Larry was a very simple and quiet guy. He would rarely show his emotions and would never get involved in an argument. Since his early days, he was fascinated by girls who were interested in some sporting activities. He believed girls are physically weak because they are not groomed in sports, right from an early age. He saw Lucy for the first time in gym picking up heavyweights. He was awed by her muscular skeleton. Lucy had seen Larry staring at her a couple of times but did not confront him as he would look away.

Once when the instructor was on leave and Lucy was lifting heavyweight on her shoulder. Lucy was struggling to put the weights down. Larry went behind her and helped her to put the weights on the ground. Larry thought she might break her back and expected Lucy to thank him but Lucy turned back and slapped Larry hard on his face. She thought he was trying to be smart. Larry with a red face turned away and went into the changing room. Another lady who was practicing daily with Lucy told her that Larry is a nice guy and a true gentleman. She knew him for a long time, and he was not like other boys. He rarely spoke to any girl in the gym. Lucy felt she had overreacted and needed to apologize. She had never apologized to anyone in her life so it was going to be very difficult for her to confront Larry. Larry with his face down and the spoiled mood was walking back when he saw Lucy coming towards him. Scared and with hand on his face to protect himself, he tried to avoid seeing her. Lucy saw his face and could not stop laughing at him. He was not what she had thought. She went and apologized to him for judging him too fast. They started meeting regularly during the gym hours and Lucy actually for the first time started looking forward to meeting a boy everyday morning. She was falling in love. Mornings increased to evening coffee shop and then parties. Lucy had never been so comfortable with any man except her father. She couldn't believe she had found such an understanding and humble person in Larry. They decided to get married. In a grand wedding function, Larry and Lucy decided to enter a wedlock. Larry's parents were not too happy with Lucy, but they didn't want to create any obstacles. Lucy's arrogant and stubborn nature would make his parents worry about their relationship. The couple had a great first year and Larry convinced Lucy to have a baby. He assured her, he would help her with parenting, and she need not worry about the child. She can continue her job post pregnancy. Larry and Lucy decided to have a baby the next year. Larry would pamper and look after her throughout the pregnancy. What she ate, what medicines she should have and when to meet her gynaecologist. All were managed by Larry meticulously. He even took the permission from the company to work part-time for six months, so he can help Lucy with raising the child.

Lucy had severe pain in the abdomen. She called up Larry who told her to rush to the hospital. He would be reaching there directly. Larry got a call from the hospital that Lucy's water bag had burst, and she was expected to deliver anytime. He was in the middle of an important work which he left immediately and rushed to the hospital. On reaching the hospital he came to know it was a baby girl. Already tired and tensed about the work he had left back in office, Larry managed to give a big smile. He was happy to hold his daughter, and the sex of the child didn't matter to him, but

Lucy felt it was because it was a girl child, he wasn't so excited. She didn't tell him anything. After meeting the child and seeing that the mother was comfortable, Larry told Lucy that he was in a middle of something very important in his office. The boss had been very considerate of him, so he wanted to go back and complete the work and would be back in an hour. Lucy allowed him to go back, but told him that she would kill him if she didn't come back on time. As she was waiting for Larry to come back. She had a doubt whether this was because it was a girl child that Larry was trying to avoid her. Would he have gone back if the child was a boy? When he came back she asked him her doubt? Larry told her to remove all this thrash from her mind. He was very happy to see the baby girl, and he always wanted a girl child. Somewhat convinced Lucy decided to let it go.

However, that wasn't true. On reaching home, Lucy was insecure for her daughter and feel that Larry was not bothered by the child. Larry was in midst of an important deal so would till late nights. This angered her more, and she felt that Larry was avoiding her daughter. Larry would do everything from changing her diapers to feeding the child. He was working part-time, so he can spend more time with her daughter. He didn't want to miss on the growth milestones of his child. He was very attached to his daughter. So whenever Lucy would question his love for his daughter he tried to avoid it in the beginning but later on, he would get angry. Lucy's insecurity for her daughter kept on growing especially when

Larry would go for overnight business trips and when he had to work overtime. She didn't want him to help her, but she wanted him to be available for her daughter all the time. This was not possible for Larry who tried to explain her many times. He even told her to go to work, and he would manage the child so that they can share the responsibilities. Lucy bluntly told him that she could not trust anyone including him. This would agitate Larry and there were frequent fights. Once when Lucy tried to accuse Larry of trying to injure her daughter when they were simply playing with toys, Larry lost it. He got angry with the accusations and told her that it was their daughter and not hers alone. Angry words turned into fights with Larry accusing Lucy of trying to bully him and dominate him. Lucy told Larry he was like other males, selfish and self-centred. She had made a big mistake by marrying him. Males like him need to be behind bars as they think females are nothing but tissues paper. Use them and throw them. Larry lost his mind and as she was arguing.

In a fit of rage Lucy who was a strong lady twisted his hand and broke his arm. Lucy thought that Larry was going to harm her. In pain and anguish, Larry could hear the bones breaking. Lucy realized what she had done. Larry called the ambulance. A case was registered against Lucy and the custody of the child was given to Larry. Larry decided not to press charges against Lucy and told the cops not to arrest her. Lucy was warned by the cops not to be around Larry and her child. Larry with tears in his eyes realized that

Lucy's behaviours were unacceptable, and she needed treatment, but he didn't dare tell her as he was scared of another confrontation. Lucy walked back from the hospital with a heavy heart. In a matter of a few minutes, life had changed. The person she loved so much had suddenly become a devil. She knew that Larry was a nice guy, but she couldn't stop herself. She decided to move to her friend place, so she can rethink what to do.

Neuroscience in recent years has determined that our fixed autonomous circuit's in the brain is actually responsible for making most of our decisions which some learned people also call it as the subconscious mind. Some connection in the neuronal circuit forms faster than the others. The receptors are more receptive to certain neurotransmitter as compared to others.
The conscious, logical and rational part of our brain, the prefrontal lobe, provides input. These circuits which have been formed by our experiences are the ultimate decision maker. Before the analysis of a particular incident is completed by the prefrontal lobe, the circuits formed by past incidents make the decisions. There are times when we feel guilty about making the wrong the decisions or choices. This is because these circuits arising from hippocampus and amygdala have already fired.
You need to know that these circuits' stores the information in the form of images and its relative emotional experiences in the hippocampus. The brain can store limited information in the form of words. The hippocampus is the part of the human

brain developed long before humans had learned a language. So when our ancestors went through a path where there was a danger to the life they stored the image and the relevant emotions relating to the incident. The next time when there was another instance of going through the same route, it alerted them, and they decided and made a conscious decision much before the analysis of the dangers involved were done. The alertness is in the form of stimulation of the hippocampal-amygdala circuit causing fear, anger or sinking feeling.

These fixed circuits are formed by taking in its consideration mostly through the visual sense, but it also pays attention to sounds, smells, emotions, kinaesthetic and proprioception (the physical sense of where you are and what's happening around you).

Remember that the job of the amygdala is to help you to survive! So it is always checking for danger. It also watches for food and sex — both important for survival, but probably not so relevant while watching a PowerPoint presentation.

These circuits let the Neo brain sort out all the verbal information.

Another interesting focus of these circuits is on novelty or change. Imagine early humans going about their day, hunting or gathering or resting in the shade after a meal. Their brain continues to scan the environment and what would they be looking for? Danger, of course!

But it wouldn't make sense to keep looking at the same thing over and over again to make sure it's safe. Instead, it is more efficient to keep an eye out for changes in your environment and then you can evaluate whether there is any danger in whatever had changed.

Another interesting part of these circuits that is that the prefrontal lobe continues to find similarities to the information it has already stored. It could be anything ranging from similar appearance, ethnicity to colour. Even with people having similar political interest makes us feel connected. Repeated reinforcement of these circuits make them autonomous and bypass the whole prefrontal circuit. People whose prefrontal lobes are not well-developed end up making more impulsive decisions based on fixed hardwired circuits.

The speed with which the thought process work is too fast for anyone to actually make a conscious decision. It solely depends upon the level of awareness and how much one does believe in the images.

The more the person is aware of this process and the related emotions the more the scope for him to rewire the fixed autonomous circuits. The level of awareness helps individual to overcome the suffering with the previous experience and helps in the formation of the new circuits. This is well explained by our teachers and parents as" act rather than react to a given situation".

Insight

The more the mind believes in the images it forms and the related past and its emotions the more the sufferings. The lesser it believes in the images it forms the more the scope for awareness and resolving difficult situations.

Lucy was exposed to female discrimination by her father. This has a horrendous effect on a child's mind. We assume that children get affected only by the words we speak and do not comprehend our body language and behaviour. This is not true.

Most of the social learning is completed in children by the age of 3 years and the rest, the children learn with experience. The images formed have a negative effect on their mind and affect their behaviours, later on. As Lucy grew up she always wanted her father to appreciate her and tried her level best to impress him. Parents are the roles models for the children in early years of their lives. However negative feedback and lack of appreciation by parent due to various reasons have a negative feedback on their mind-set.

They lose their confidence and end up being pessimist. Children whose parents give a lot of negative feedback end complaining more often for silly reason and refuse to take responsibility. There is also evidence of increased self-doubt in children where parents have a habit of frequent fault-finding in children. This is followed by a vicious loop of confrontation in the teenage life.

As Lucy grew up, she became a sports trainer and had a good physique. The marks her father had created by the discrimination had an effect on her married life.

The brain would go into automation with the simplest hint of gender discrimination. This would create a turmoil and Lucy would experience all the emotion she had experienced. Lucy would overreact and fight back as she was a strong girl now.

This was happening at such a fast pace without her knowledge that she did not realize what the opposite person was thinking. We tend to overreact in difficult situation. The reason being defending ourselves from the same bitter experience rather than attacking the other for their fault, with our words and at times action.

In most of the cases like in Lucy there is not much active awareness of the given situation.

Lucy needed to break these chain of events and not get carried away with the belief and assumption that her husband would do the same with his daughter. This could have been possible only by being aware and putting the agitated mind at rest.

The advice given by father to cultivate compassion and empathy is another way where we can understand other people's point of view and be emotionally intelligent. But it is not easy for her to break these automated neurons of mistrust from firing.

Lucy dejected with what had happened moved to her friend's place as she wanted to be away from all the negative thoughts. She was not the person who would think much about her actions. She always believed however you react is always the best for you. But this time the sinking feeling was not leaving her. She was missing her husband and her child. She knew that she could not live without them. She tried training, but she would burst out in tears even with a little noise around her. She didn't like being so emotionally driven but her feelings seemed to be dominating her mind. She knew something must be done before it gets too late. The noise in her mind, the pain in her heart was different from that she had ever experienced. She was feeling helpless and that was making her feel more depressed.

She knew Larry loved her and that she had been too harsh on him. Lucy knew Larry had always respected her and stood by him in her difficult times. Unlike her father, Larry was supportive both in helping her raise the child and in her professional decisions. In fact, people in her workplace were jealous of her as she had such an understanding husband. Lucy did not know how to control the negative thought and doubts she was getting. As she lay down trying to do her shoulder press in her gym, tears rolled down her eyes. She realized she had made a blunder in the way she had behaved. Sobbing she went in the park staring at the kids playing in the park with their father. She missed her father. She remembered her father's last words" Whenever

your life is difficult and you are feeling helpless
and there are no solutions you can see…always
remember that everything in the world comes
back if you cultivate compassion and empathy for
people". She decided to give it a try. She started
first helping her students and guiding them rather
than forcing them or humiliating them, which she
used to do. The students were pleasantly surprised
and started sharing their problems. Lucy found it
difficult initially and would get annoyed. But she
was determined to give her father's advice a
thorough effort. More and more students started
training with her and Lucy realized the change.
She decided to give it a shot with Larry. She went
to meet Larry although she was strictly forbidden
by the cops. She knocked at the door with
trembling hands. Larry opened the door and was
angry at seeing Lucy. He started shouting at her
and told her to go away. Lucy simply stood there
with tears in her eyes requested Larry to hear her
out. She promised Larry she will never come back
again but wanted him to give her a chance to
explain. Larry had never seen Lucy like this. He
called her in. Lucy told Larry why she had
behaved like a moron. Her experiences, her
childhood memories and how she had changed
her behaviour in her gym. She apologized to
Larry for being so inconsiderate and a bad wife.
Larry was shocked at seeing Lucy apologizing. It
was difficult for him to understand this change.
He couldn't believe his eyes. He realized that she
had changed and decided to give her a chance. He
hugged her and told her that he was always with
her and next time he will not to give her a chance

to complain. He would run away before breaking his hand. Lucy knew the real difficulty had now started, but she decided that she will trust her husband and try to talk to him whenever there are any differences rather than react. In a couple of weeks, Lucy became calm and could let go of her unwarranted suspicions. She still was the same strong girl but now she would understand people's emotions and would try to reason out before simply judging people. As Lucy lied on her bed in Larry's arms she realized that however James, her father had behaved with her in her childhood, the last few words of James saved her marriage and probably her life. She forgave him and decided to move on.

<u>8.</u>

Moses

In our pursuit to mix automation with awareness we have developed from part of the creation to so-called rulers of creation in the journey, we have migrated from being a part of stillness of nature to the slayers of our own peace and tranquillity.

As Sam was trying to remember the names of any old friend he had missed, he could not recollect the name, one of his friend who was a genius and the topper in his high school. His wife Jane had seen his interview a couple of times, but she couldn't recollect his name. They decided to find the name and number of his friend who was the director of a multinational global company running cake shops across the globe. He was awarded as the most dynamic businessman and his company was listed in Forbes 100 that year." Voila! His name is Moses" Jane exclaimed. They found out his number from the directory.
Actually, Moses was a common friend of both Jane and Sam. Both knew him well and Sam always had a doubt that Moses had a secret crush on Jane, but he never told them.
Jane called up Moses's Office and told the operator she wanted to speak to Moses. The operator told her to give her name and what she wanted to speak to him about, so she can convey

her message. Jane gave her the details and waited patiently for him to come online. It was nearly thirty minutes when Sam told Jane that there was no point in waiting as Moses was a big man, and he wouldn't want to speak to commoners like them. She was about to hang up when a loud but friendly voice on the phone said "hey Jane. How are you? Do you still miss me?" It was Moses on the line. Jane spoke to him for some time and then handed over the phone to Sam. Moses spoke very politely to Sam over the phone and accepted the invitation to come to the party. Sam was surprised at how Moses voice had toned down and was very polite now. Moses was an arrogant boy in the school and rarely used to talk to everyone. He would never get into an unnecessary conversation on hobbies or entertainment as he considered them to be a waste of time. He was a perfectionist right from the early age and was very straight and direct in his conversations. He didn't believe in greeting or having friendly chitchats as they would simply waste his time. He would always tell everyone that every word coming out of our mouth must have a purpose. Sam could feel that his tone and behaviours had changed. He thought as we grow up we all change our behaviour so must have Moses. But every one of us has a story. What must be his story?

Moses was born into an affluent family. His father was a navy officer. Since his childhood days, Moses had a habit of being organized. Discipline and being organized were the two word which had a great influence on his life. Moses had always been a good student and there were rarely any instances when the teacher had called his mother to school. There was one thing Moses had missed in his childhood that his father never allowed him to see television. He always believed that it was a waste of time and it is for civilians who had no purpose in their life. There was always a craving in Moses mind for screen time as he would feel out of the place, when friends used to discuss about sitcom they saw the day before. Moses had imagined most of the characters as the friends described them but never saw them on the screen. Young Moses used to feel that his father was behaving like dictator, forcing his views on him.

The big Hoardings of Simpson or Superman were just restricted to large big banners on the road or magazines in Moses life. As Moses turned 16 years he would secretly go to cinemas or plays. He was fascinated by new gadgets as they came into the market. This was the time when computers and laptops had just come in the Market and the world had started getting digitalized. He would bunk school and go and watch movies. This started affecting his studies and one day his father came to know about his bunking and declining grades. Now Moses was 16 years he was not scared of his father. There was a huge fight with his father that night and Moses decided to leave the house. He quit his studies. He started looking for a job and found it at a nearby bakery. He stayed at the bakery in the night and worked during the daytime. He would go to a nearby electronic shop and would watch television from the glass outside. He vowed to himself that he will one day purchase the best gadgets in the world. He worked in the bakery for a couple of years and finally decided to start his small bakery shop with the money he had collected. He rented a place and started making fancy cakes in his shop. Slowly he became popular and he got a bigger shop. He would sit on the computer researching different ways he can decorate and add flavours to the cake.

His bakery business turned into a Cake shop in a few years. He started hiring employees as his business flourished. He decided to open more branches as the demand grew. He would experiment with new flavours as he gained popularity. Any new flavour in any part of the world would first be seen at Moses cake shop. He had around 10 branches by the end of three years. He realized if he had to grow he must come up with a better idea. He decided to go online. He looked for new investors and decided to increase more branches throughout the country. Moses cakes shop was the first online cake shop in the country with over 1000 branches all over the country. His workforce was around 10000 employees. Being a tech-savvy, Moses was spending most of his time either on the computer or laptop or for a presentation for the workplace. Except for business-related, he would rarely have a conversation with anyone. He had never had any serious relationships. Although he had a few casual affairs or one-night stand he was never involved in any serious relationship. He missed his mother whom he would call up but hated his father because he felt that he had ruined his life. Moses was a highly successful entrepreneur and had received many awards and laurels. He was named as the most promising entrepreneur of the year.

He wanted to make his company global, so he decided to take over other regional companies which were not doing so well. One such company which had a good presence in Europe but was running in losses. He decided to meet the CEO and give her an offer she could not refuse. Her name was Betty who had inherited the business from her father. It was doing relatively well but after her father passed away she found it difficult to handle as she was a fashion designer. The company was running in deep loses and Betty was tired of the calls from the lenders. Betty was inexperienced and used to take her younger brother for all meetings. That day when the meeting between Betty and Moses was scheduled, her younger brother didn't turn up as he had some submission in college. As Betty entered the room she saw a middle-aged man with a serious look on his face. Betty was a jovial girl and never understood why business guys have to keep such a serious expression on their face. As the meeting progressed Moses's personal assistant started briefing about his companies profile to Betty. Betty saw Moses face, and she burst out laughing seeing him so serious, when the assistant was actually been talking about his company. She excused herself, and then she told Moses directly that she had already mailed him about the assets and liabilities of the company and also what was the expected amount she planned to sell her company. Moses told Betty that the company was loss-making and that nobody would ever invest in such a company. He was gracious enough to come and it would be a fool who would buy this company. These were the tactics used by Moses to bargain and get a good deal. He offered her half the amount of money that she had quoted. She thought for a while. This was the only buyer she had got in the last six months, and she had no choice. She agreed to sign the deal with the amount Moses quoted. Moses had a grin on his face. He had got the deal for much lesser amount than he had thought. As the meeting got over and the paperwork was done, Moses tapped on Betty's shoulder. "I would like to give you advice. Never ever do business as he had fooled her into buying the company in a much lesser amount than what it was worth."

Betty turned back and gave him a smile." I know that the company is worth much more, but she was happy as she had made the right decision as she had no choice in the given circumstances. You are partially right, Sir. I am laughing even after making a loss and there is no smile on your face even after getting a good deal. So who is a fool? "She added. Betty's answer stung Moses like a thorn. For the next two days, he would rehearse how to smile in front of the mirror. He realized he hardly smiled in the entire day. He was scheduled for the final meeting with Betty the next day. Moses felt a strange emptiness in his heart. This girl had really disturbed his peace of mind. He wanted to prove it to her he could be happy. When Moses entered the room and saw Betty, he tried hard not to look serious. He looked around casually as if he was least bothered. His assistant could not understand why his boss was behaving strangely. Betty couldn't stop laughing at Moses behaving like a jerk. Moses got angry at Betty and told her," why are you laughing now? Can't you see I am not looking serious?" Moses exploded. The entire room burst out laughing including Moses. He was caught unaware, but he was surprised he felt happy at seeing Betty laughing instead of getting annoyed at her. Moses for the first time decided to change the amount and give her the right amount she deserved. He told Betty that he knew why he was not able to smile after the deal and thanked her for making him realize it.

They started meeting regularly, sometimes at the coffee shop and sometimes at movies. Moses stopped sitting with gadgets and like teenagers would spend hours talking to Betty on the phone. In his quest for growing his company, he had forgone his youth. Moses suddenly had a new meaning to his boring life. He knew he was in love and would sing songs for Betty. Betty would laugh at him and told him he was the worst singer she had ever met. Betty's cheerful nature started influencing Moses behaviours. People at work would love it when he would come to their table and ask them how they had been that weekend. Moses was a changed man. Betty and Moses got married in the church and had twins by the second year. Both were beautiful boys and were very lucky for Moses. His company was listed in the

Forbes 100 top companies which were once his target. As the boys turned 2 and there were new entrants in the cake industry. There was stiff competition and Moses would stay more at the office. He had suffered a minor loss as he was not focusing on work like he used to before the birth of the kids. He would sit down in front of the laptop throughout the day. In a couple of months, the problem was dealt with, and he was not facing any current issue. He was hooked up to gadgets like before. Even at home he would be either be on the mobile or the laptop. Betty could see he was not working but would be simply surfing the sites.

Moses did not even know which class his kids were studying or what they were doing even when at home. They had not been on vacations for the last 6 years. Moses would hardly spend time at home although Betty would keep updating him whenever he was home. He would come late at night and would leave early in the morning. His kids were the only children in school whose father never came for their annual functions. Moses, only excuses was there was work pressure, and he would try to make it next time. Moses at times realized this but something or other would come up. Once when Moses was trying to sneak in late at night, both his sons were waiting at the door to talk to him. His son Rubin and Zain wanted Moses to come for a soccer match with them the next day. They didn't want to go with Betty alone. Moses was tired. He tried to give them lame excuses. But the kids didn't buy his excuse. They wanted him to promise them that if he didn't turn up they would not eat food that day. Moses shouted at Betty who was sleeping and was not aware of the late father-son conversation. He got angry and threatened the two 8-year-old kids with dire consequences. The boys got scared and started crying out loudly. Moses tried to pacify them. But the kids were in no mood to listen. The problem was that Moses had to fly away for a big business meeting on the next day and would not be able to reach for the soccer match. The boys started throwing things at Moses who lost his temper and pushed Rubin on the sofa. Rubin lost his balance and hit his head against the table. Blood started pouring from his head. Betty who was asleep got up after hearing all the commotion. She was shocked at on seeing Rubin cry, with blood all over his face. Moses panicked and was froze, Betty picked him up and rushed to the hospital. She told Moses not to enter the hospital room. Moses could not believe what he had done. Betty took the kids after the stitches were done, to her parents' house. She had been tolerating Moses's behaviours from a long time, but she couldn't anymore. She decided to leave him. She registered a complaint against him and Moses was warned not to be around his kids. Moses was alone in his house. He couldn't believe what had happened. He picked up his smartphone and threw it on the wall. He hadn't realized he had become a machine while being around machines. A week later one morning he got a mail from the postman. Betty had filed for a divorce. Moses was heartbroken. His whole life had come to a standstill.

*We have discussed before how our minds and most of the creations work in automation. Although we are born with only a few automation which we have inherited or are related to our experience. But as the experiences become deep-rooted, our brain tends to be more inclined to this automation. The brain tends to associate the newer experiences with the previous ones and reinforce the formed pathway. One of the primary reasons that people find it difficult to form new pathways or ideas at a later stage is basically because of the inherent ability of the neurons to move in automation. This automation also has a very big role in the evolution of mankind. These are the automation which is responsible for humans performing a complicated task like driving a car or making a mobile. If it weren't for us gaining through the past inventions, we would never be able to improvise and make more complicated gadgets. The biggest example is the "**Evolution of smartphone**" passing through a series of automation from the typewriter to the computer, laptop, notebook and finally the smartphone. We can find the effect of automation even in the construction of buildings, vehicles or machines. Languages are the simplest example of automation which made these complex inventions possible. But was this simply possible with automation in the brain? The answer is no. If people had stopped being aware of the limitations of the computer there wouldn't have been any new inventions like laptop or smartphones. This awareness was the reason* *along with automation which created newer and faster vehicles. You can see any technological advances in mankind and you will realize that awareness mixed with automation was the prime reason which made our lives today much easier than our ancestors. But these crucial mixture has also had its impact on mankind. Not only did the neurons function in automation so did the emotions associated with the experiences. When we are on a train or airplane what gives us happiness and fright is our previous emotion associated with our experience. Advances in technology should have decreased our stress and made our life easier, but this has actually contributed an increase of our worries and the associated stress.*

Another reason is the need for social interaction which is responsible for our behaviours and how we engage with people. This has today become the most sought out skill although the advance in technology seems to be moving at lightning speed in the recent times. This untamed amygdala and poor regulation by the prefrontal lobe result in impulsive behaviours and reactions. Increased aggressiveness and competitiveness in a complex world has created havoc. Survival of fittest which was once a gradual self-limiting statement, where nature had its own way of playing fair with all beings has been replaced today with a more selfish and complex human psychology.

Insight

Whenever, any restriction is placed on a human mind, there is a natural tendency to be curious about it. This is a case with most of the things in our life. The moment you are diagnosed with Diabetes, there is natural inclination to have more sugar laden food. Our mind doesn't like restrictions and rules. But without them our lives and society, in general, would be chaotic.

Moses was not allowed to see television and his father kept him away from screen, but this created an enhanced curiosity in Moses, leading to an uncontrollable urge. The main purpose of technology is to make things easy for human life. This has shifted now to entertainment and at times distraction from our everyday daily stressful activities.

Moses became rebellious, like most kids do, when restrictions are put on them. In the recent years there is a big burst of new gadgets with frequent-changing technology. Moses decided to leave the house after a confrontation with his father. He was lucky to get job and his creative mind was able to grow his business many folds.

He used technology for his growth. We all realize that most of the business flourish online and my book would have been read by you if it weren't for the burst of new technology in the last decade. His attraction got him glued to the gadgets and his interaction with people reduced many folds. This creates a void in human brain. Too much of screen time causes people to be more aggressive and insensitive.

Using a gadget frequently reduces the work done by our brain and this leads our active thinking brain to be lazy.

His urge from his childhood compounded by the stress of losing business made Moses more aggressive. Many do not realize the need of the brain for social engagement and are too dependent on gadget. This ends up leading to confrontations with family and friends. However, being away from technology, is also not a viable option. Striking a balance between screen time and fruitful engaging conversation is the only way we can prevent the harmful effects.

Moses need to be aware of these effects and convince his family that he will give them adequate time. This would be beneficial for both him and his family. That would happen only if Zarine forgives him, for hitting their children, which is difficult for any mother.

Moses's family troubles were having an impact on his work. He was losing his temper at a drop of the hat. The sales were suffering and the shares had fallen. The investors were losing their patience on him. Moses would sit on his chair and would consume alcohol from morning to evening. He had stopped using the fancy phones which he had always fantasized. The simplest noise of a television playing in the background would make him lose his temper. Moses divorce was in the final stages. Moses had willingly agreed to give

the custody of their children to Betty, and she had
refused to take any alimony from him. Betty had
taken up the job as a fashion designer in a
renowned company. As Moses was walking
towards the courtroom, drunk and supported by
his assistant? He fell down and hurt his head.
Betty who had been watching him ran towards
him. As blood oozed out of the abrasion on his
forehead. Betty watched with empathy at her
husband. Moses opened his eyes and looked at
Betty, "I am sorry Betty for making your life
horrible. I am guilty of spoiling your life and my
kid's life. But there was nobody except you who
could have made a difference in my life. You
were the reason why I was alive. Life will not be
worth it without you in my life. I am transferring
all my wealth and property to you and will never
come back but please do not divorce me. At least
let me die peacefully with a wife and children
rather than being alone as I had always lived."
Betty saw the grief and remorse in Moses' eyes.
She walked away leaving Moses in the
courtroom. She couldn't believe the same Moses
who had once been such a dynamic person had
today become a weak person. She thought about
her kids.
The next day she went to Moses's house. Moses
opened the door and invited her in. She asked him
whether he will change and try to be a better
father and husband if she came back. How can
she be sure that he will not revert to his old habits
and behaviours? Moses smiled and handed over
the papers. He told her that she now owned
everything, so she could throw him out anytime.

Betty was convinced and hugged him. She forgave him for his mistakes. She decided to give him another chance as the kids would be missing their father after the divorce. Moses with tears in his eyes told her that once again she made him understand how to live with a smile on his face. His family was the reason for his smile. The divorce proceedings were withdrawn and Moses decided not to get work to his house. He would spend time with the family and cut down on his work. He would attend all the school functions with his kids. Moses would spend at least 1 month in a year with the family and go on a vacation. And he would switch off his phones when on a trip. On one such vacation Moses looked lovingly at his wife and told her now I have understood that **"Man-made machines to smile and when a machine starts making a man smile, your life goes away."**

9.

Kim

The more we are aware of these automations in the mind, the lesser fuel we give to these brain pathways to become rigid and fixed. The more fixed and rigid our thinking, the lesser we are in control of our behaviours and reactions.

Sam was very excited about the party. He wanted Jane to meet all the people with whom he had spent time before she came in his life. Jane mocked Sam that, "she was jealous, already after seeing his excitement. Sam told her that, to wait when he sees Kim who was a year older than her. Last he heard was that, she was a successful model. Sam realized that he had not called her. After making a few calls to his old mates, he was able to get her phone number. Sam wondered, whether Kim would be able to recognize the shy boy, who had once been her date for the prom. He called her and asked her, whether she recognized him. Kim thought for the moment and suddenly recalled. "It's the boy who had won the bet, and she had a wonderful time with him in the prom". Sam was happy that she still remembered him. He invited her to the party, which she readily agreed. As soon as Kim hung up, she recollected the good olden days. Life had taken a sudden twist and her life had changed. As she sat down sipping a cup of coffee, the bell rang. She pressed the remote on

her automatic wheelchair and opened the door.
Her son had come home from school. She
thanked God that she was blessed with a very
caring son who never made her realize, she was
disabled. Kim wished, she had been this humble
and calm before.
Kim was always a pampered child from birth. Her
father Brian would fulfil all her wishes after his
bitter divorce from Kim's mom. Kim was 12
years when the couple separated after a very bitter
custody battle. Kim's mom, Veronica was an
alcoholic and the court had given a ruling, that
Kim was safe with her father. This decision did
not go down well with little Kim, and she used to
miss her mother. Brian tried his level best, but he
was unable to pacify his daughter. So Brian
decided to marry his office colleague Mia who
was actually the reason why Brian had a divorce.
Brian was having an affair with Mia which
Veronica came to know after 4 years. She started
confronting Brian about the affair which he
always denied. She had caught Brian many a
time, but he would always give some lame
excuse. This was the period when Kim's mom got
addicted to alcohol. She would look at Kim and
decided to keep the family intact for her sake.
Kim, on the other hand, would see her mom
crying in the middle of the night.
This went on for a year but what happened next
was intolerable for her. Veronica had to go to her
parents place, as her mom was not doing well. It
was a one-hour travel from where Kim used to
stay. She had called up Brian and informed him
that she would be coming the next morning.

When she was unpacking the clothes she realized she had forgotten to carry her tax papers, which she had to be filed the next day. It was the last day, and she had to submit them. She realized she was not carrying any copy and had to go back home in the night. Her mother was doing better now. Veronica knew that if she left early, she would be able to reach her house before midnight. With little Kim sleeping in the rear seat, Veronica rushed back home. There was a lot of traffic on the highway. She tried to call up Brian but his phone was not reachable. As she reached home way past midnight, there was a car parked outside her door. Worried about her husband she woke up Kim and rushed into the house. The showpieces in the living room were scattered and room was messy. The sofa had been shifted to the side. As the mother-daughter duo entered the house, they got scared that Brian was in some danger and a robber had entered the house. Veronica picked up the stick behind the door and entered in her room. Since it was late in the night there was absolute silence. It was dark in her room. Veronica switched on the light and was shocked to see Mia lying naked next to Brian. Veronica put her hands on Kim's eyes. Her suspicion about his affair had come true. She was shocked at seeing Brian like this. She left the room with her daughter crying out loudly. Kim couldn't believe Brian had broken her trust. Hurt and angry with herself, Veronica left the house. She decided to divorce him. She found it difficult to manage her emotions for a few days, but she gradually started working and accepting the situation. Even when

she lost the custody of her child, Veronica
accepted the fate and wished her daughter a good
health and life. All this had a very negative
impact on Kim. She could not forget her mother's
expression when they had entered her room. Brian
got married to Mia so that he could look after
Kim as she was growing up. Kim never accepted
her as her mother. She would spend a lot of time
with her friends and avoided any interaction with
Mia. The only person she spoke to was her father.
Brian would never say no to his daughter. Kim
turned out to be a beautiful lady just like her
mother. She did not believe in relationship and
would always believe that relationships were
weaknesses, which everyone must avoid. She had
many boyfriends in her school and all her affairs
were casual. At times, she would be in more than
one relationship. One such incident was when she
had a bet with her boyfriend that she could go out
with any geek for the prom. Sam happened to
enter the room at the same time. She asked him
for a date. Sam could not believe his luck, and so
this is how Sam and Kim met each other. Soon,
after the prom, Sam came to know about the bet.
He was hurt but he also called himself lucky. Kim
meanwhile got a modelling contract with a
company. She completed it by going to high
school in the morning and finishing her modelling
assignments in the evening. As time went by she
was offered more and more projects. As she
excelled in her career, her woes of having long-
term relationship continued. She would always
feel lonely. She had everything that a young girl
of her age could wish for except a companion

whom she could trust. Kim was featured in many magazines and was a popular artist. In terms of earning, she earned a decent income through her photo shoots and advertisements. In spite of her having many friends she was unable to trust people. She always felt that the person would cheat on her. This would create a defensive attitude in her towards any close relationship. She believed before the opposite person would ditch her and hurt her emotions, she would dump the guy and show him his place. This would create a lot of loneliness in her.

As she climbed the ladder of her career she became more and more lonely. This was until Jonathan came into her life. Jonathan was a freelance photographer, whom Kim had met during a photo-shoot. He was a tall man of around 6 feet with broad shoulders and masculine physique. He had been known for his creativity and was one of the most respected photographers for his unique work by the producers. Jonathan was a calm person who recently had come out of a broken marriage. His wife had dumped him for a young boy and this had made Jonathan very upset. He would not talk to anybody on the sets. It was the first time in Kim's shoot that Jonathan was the photographer. Kim was very particular about the angle, the light and the expression which the photographer shot. She would interfere and at times fight with the photographer on the sets, if things were not according to her liking. It so happened that, while shooting Kim did not like the angles which Jonathan was shooting from. She suggested him some angles which would have a better output. Jonathan chose to ignore her advice and went on with his work. Soon after the shoot when Kim saw the photographs she realized Jonathan did not listen to her. She fumed with anger and told the producer to throw the photographer out of the room. She started abusing Jonathan and told him that, "he was just a photographer, and he should never forget that." Everybody who knew Jonathan personally felt sorry for him. But nobody dared speak against Kim who was famous for throwing a tantrum on the set. Jonathan quietly listened to Kim's harsh words and left the set without responding to her. Kim convinced the producer to get another photographer and reshoot the event. The next day the new photographer did as Kim told. The angles, the light, and the changes were all edited by Kim. Finally, when the photographs came in the evening Kim saw the photographs on screen and told him, what a fool Jonathan was. You can see that these have come out so good. Everyone agreed to what she was saying. Nobody wanted to ruffle her feathers. But as she was leaving, the spot boy came and told her the truth. The photographs she was seeing were shot by Jonathan and the producer had already discarded the ones shot by the second photographer. He also told about Jonathan's personal life tragedy. On hearing this Kim felt horrible. She had behaved unfairly with Jonathan. She wanted to make up, so she decided to go and meet him. With a bouquet, she reached his residence, she found that it was locked. The neighbours told her that he might be by the seashore nearby as he normally spends a lot of time there. On reaching the sea shore she saw a man playing with little street kids'. On coming close she realized that it was Jonathan. She was amazed to find him happy and running around. She apologized to Jonathan for her behaviours and asked him to come for a coffee. Jonathan told her that he had already forgiven her, and he was lucky to have a date with a beautiful model like her. They started enjoying each other's company and would meet up every day. This was the first time Kim had told somebody about her mother and how she missed her. How she felt dreadful living with her stepmom Mia whom she held responsible for ruining her parent's life. Kim also told him about her problem in relationships. She was getting attracted to Jonathan, in turn, Jonathan wanted someone to get over his wife. The friendship grew into love and love finally led to their marriage. They were perfectly made for each other. Kim with her aggressive and impulsive behaviour and Jonathan with his calmness and cool-headed made an ideal couple. Kim realized that she finally found her soul mate. She knew she could trust Jonathan. They had a handsome son one year after marriage. Everything was beautiful and Jonathan was very supportive. She had lost her post-pregnancy weight and Jonathan used to help her work out and get her fitness back. She got her figure back just in six months and was modelling again. Life was beautiful for Kim and Jonathan. "Until! That unfortunate day", Kim remembered. Kim and Jonathan were invited to a party where top producers and models were going to come.

Kim was looking beautiful and as they arrived at the party the journalist as usual surrounded, Kim trying to take her interview. Jonathan was left alone with his son. As they entered the ballroom, Laila who was a young model around 25 years came next to Jonathan and started talking to him. Kim who had finished her interview saw Jonathan talking to Laila. Jonathan introduced Laila as a model whose photographs he had shot a couple of days back. Laila asked Kim if it was okay if she danced with Jonathan. Kim felt uncomfortable but nodded. She expected Jonathan to turn down the offer. Jonathan took her hand and danced with her in the ballroom for some time. Burning with jealousy, she snatched Jonathan's hand and started dancing with him. For the whole party, Kim was staring at Laila feeling insecure and overtly jealous. As they were driving back home, Kim and Jonathan had a fight, and she told him to not take a photo-shoot with Laila again. Kim felt that Laila was stalking Jonathan. She was right to an extent. Laila was a newcomer, and she was using Jonathan to get new contracts. Jonathan agreed that he will not recommend her to anyone or shoot with her again. Things were fine between the couple for a couple of days. Once when Jonathan was taking a bath, Kim read a whatsapp message from Laila. She wrote that she was missing him and wanted to meet him. Kim got angry and confronted Jonathan. But Jonathan said that, he has not spoken to her, since that day. Kim was not ready to believe him, and she stormed out of the room. Jonathan explained to her to trust

him, and he would never cheat on
her. Laila would keep sending messages in spite
of Jonathan telling her that he didn't want to
speak to her. After a week when Jonathan was
doing a photo-shoot, Kim decided to surprise him
by coming to the sets. As Jonathan finished his
shoot suddenly two hands came on his eyes and
blindfolded him. He recognized the soft hands
and called out "darling it's a nice surprise". He
turned around and saw it was Laila. Jonathan was
expecting Kim to be there and was shocked to
see Laila. From the corner of his eye, he saw Kim
who had just entered. Jonathan froze like a statue.
Surprisingly Kim didn't say a word. Jonathan
tried to explain but Kim told her we will talk
later. Angry and hurt Kim told Jonathan to come
with him. The images of her father with Mia
flashed in front of her eyes. She thought Jonathan
was cheating on her just like Veronica, her
mother. As Jonathan drove, Kim started accusing
him of cheating on him Jonathan tried to explain
but Kim thought that he was two-timing her. Just
then the phone rang and Jonathan picked up the
phone. Kim saw the name on the screen.
It was Laila. She snatched the phone from
Jonathan's hand and as Jonathan turned to tell her
to calm down, the car rammed into a speeding
truck. Kim lost her consciousness. It was a major
accident where the entire front part, especially the
driver's seat was completely destroyed. Jonathan
died on the spot itself. Kim was taken to the
intensive care unit and went into a coma. She
regained consciousness after 20 days. When she
opened her eyes she realized she had lost both her

legs. She was also told that Jonathan was no more. This was very tragic and Kim was inconsolable. She wanted to kill herself. But then a little voice told her, "Mama I missed you". It was her son and the purpose for her to be alive. She wondered how she will raise him without her legs. She felt dejected and depressed.

As we grow older we strengthen our old pathways. Connecting it newer incidents we keep on making the old one's pathways fixed and more rigid. At times these pathways which represent the thought processes become autonomous. Let me explain what I mean by autonomous thought processes. At times, we react to a given incident without making any effort or having any voluntary say over it. Later on, we regret saying something offensive or reacting in a way which we absolutely do not believe it. We call it impulsive behaviour but the real reason is these autonomous pathways are moving without any voluntary say. This is also termed by many as having the subconscious mind as discussed before which we cannot control or modulate. There will be endless occasions in every individual's life, when we know by our logical reasoning that there is something wrong in the way we behave but the brain makes the decision so swiftly that before the amygdala-prefrontal circuits are operational, the amygdala has already sent the messages to the respective motor circuits.

Although being aware of these circuits post the incident does give us the insights into what is right and wrong, but it needs a greater degree of awareness to overcome the autonomous circuits.

Insight

Kim from birth was a pampered child. She had seen the bitter divorce of her parents and always blamed her stepmom for separating them. This had created a negative and brittle image of relationships in her mind. She was always insecure in committing in a relationship as she had the fear that this would cause her more pain. These events had a mark on young Kim's mind, and she had many failed relationships. Her career in modelling gave the necessary self-confidence but her self-esteem was always low. Self-confidence is what people think about you and self-esteem is what you think about yourself.

The insecurity in relationships and fear of the pain arising from a failed relationship had created a fixed automation that 'relationship always fails'. She had many failed relationship until she met Jonathan. Even with Jonathan, the process of being insecure of the other models didn't stop. She kept on ruminating about an imaginary relationship which never existed between her husband and Laila. Most of the times when we are caught on the web of these fixed thoughts, we are unable to see the real situation. Ruminating about an imaginary affair of a spouse is one of the reasons of friction between some couples, which many times, end in a divorce.

Kim was unable to control her behaviour. She ended up destroying her life by letting her emotional brain (amygdala) go on a rampage.

The guilt of her husband's death with the responsibility of raising her son is a difficult situation for most of us to **come back**. The way forward is to calm things down, introspect and find a resolution to her problems. Since modelling was the only thing she knew, she would have to explore new professions and talents rather than sulking and cursing her destiny. This wouldn't be possible until she calms down the noise in her mind.

Kim was thinking how she will raise her child when she is not even able to get up on her legs. How will she earn money and who will give her a job? She had formally passed only high school, and she didn't know anything except modelling. She was discharged from the hospital. Although she had a maid and a cook she realized she needs to get independent and start working before she finishes of all her reserve money in the bank. Just then an advertisement for a new foldable electronic chair with remote came flashing of the television. This was Kim was looking for. She bought the chair which could go up and down and move in all directions. She could reach the kitchen shelf and cook food. So one problem was solved. She needed to find a job. She saw Jonathan's old camera and gadgets. Kim realized that they were of no use to her. So she called up one of her producers who offered her a decent price. She boarded a taxi and took her foldable chair. She reached the shooting unit she saw a photo-shoot of a model. As soon as she went close by she realized it was Laila. She felt a rush of anger in her body. With her fists closed she wanted to tell Laila that it was because of her, her life was ruined. But just then the thought of the accident and Jonathan's last words telling her to calm down passed through her mind. She realized it was this anger and jealousy which had cost Jonathan's life. She calmed herself down and saw the photo shoot. The producer was not satisfied with the photo-shoot. Something was missing. Kim realized the light was dull, so she prompted the producer to increase the brightness. Laila's face needed to be turned more towards the right side. Kim prompted the producer what were the changes needed to be done. She had a good experience of production when she was shooting. The photographer took the photographs. The producer was extremely satisfied with the output and the shooting was over. Kim's knowledge of production impressed the producer and offered her an assistant producer's job. She readily accepted it. The producer asked her to hand over the camera she had got. Kim refused politely by saying that she needed to do more with the camera and had got the answers to her questions. She looked at Laila and called her. Kim apologized to her for her behaviours. She told her she was very beautiful and one day will become a supermodel.

10.

Georgina

Awareness is a habit difficult to cultivate because of man's greed for social interactions.

As the date for the party was coming closer, Sam had this weird feeling that he was forgetting someone. He was excited to meet his old friends partly because of Anna and her rescue story, but he also he wanted to show everyone the positive changes in his behaviour. He was no longer that geek or shy boy as he was in high school. Sam came home after work, he asked Anna where her mother was. Anna replied that she had called, and told that she would be late. Sam was wondering that the office shuts by six pm and it was around 9 pm, Jane should be home. Sam didn't want to assume or react, so he decided to wait for some time. The doorbell rang and Sam was relieved that Jane was back from work. After freshening up, Jane came to the dinner table. She told Sam that she had met their friend Georgina. Sam knew her because she was Tom's cousin sister. What did Jane not know that Sam had a brief affair with Georgina in high school-days? It lasted for a week but Sam realized that Georgina was not his type of girl. He never told Jane about it because he didn't give it that much importance. He just took it is as a causal relationship. When Sam heard about Georgina, he told Jane about the brief relationship he had with Georgina. Jane was shocked and told Sam that this was the weirdest thing about Sam she had heard since her marriage. She couldn't believe how a guy like Sam could enter a relationship with a fickle minded girl like Georgina. Although she had drastically changed, now in her college days she was extremely fickle minded and would keep changing her boyfriend's just on the basis of public opinions. She had invited her, as Georgina would regularly ask for help to make certain decisions in her life, and they both shared their notes. Jane couldn't stop laughing at Sam who started getting embarrassed. Jane excused herself and told him about Georgina and her ever-changing seasons.

Georgina was born in a most reserved and conservative Jewish family. Right from school-days, her decisions were always taken by her mother. Mother would never ask her, what she wanted or does have any choice or liking. Till she was 10 there was no problem but as she grew up, she had her own choices but her mother would give negative feedback to the child and depress her. She would ultimately be convinced after listening to the criticism and would give up. This created a lot of indecisiveness in her, and she would always ask her mother for everything. Even which friends were good and which were bad for her was decided by her mom. Once when a boy proposed her when she was 13, she told the boy, she will ask her mother and then reply to him the next day. Everyone in school came to know about it, and they would tease Georgina. Georgina turned out to be a beautiful girl with long black hair. She was average in her studies and wanted to be an architect. Her mother was diagnosed with a fatal ovarian cancer which was in the final stage. She died within 6 months of her diagnosis. This had a major effect on Georgina who was completely dependent on her mother for decision-making in her life. It was like a computer without a CPU. She found it extremely difficult to even buy butter. She couldn't decide which brand to buy? Soon, she was lonely, as her father who was a captain in a ship was rarely home. She would speak to everyone in the neighbourhood and take their advice for her confusions. Georgina felt lonely as they were nobody in the house except her. She hated staying in the house and night would be the most dreadful time of the day, when she was alone. Most of the times, she would feel comfortable when she was around people. Georgina would take peoples advice for trivial matters and would blindly follow them without actually using her mind. This would create a lot of confusion, and she would end up buying multiple brands of the same product. This lack of confidence or decision-making ability also reflected in her relationship. She would have multiple boyfriends and would date boys at the same time. The most common argument she gave was that she liked someone's eyes or their muscles. Every boy had some talent, and she couldn't make up her mind whom to stay with. Once she did get seriously involved about a boy and was about to marry him. But the boy came to know that she was two-timing him and was also dating another boy. He dumped her. This incident left a deep scar in her mind, and she decided not to get so serious about any boy. Her affair with Sam was during that period. She simply stopped liking him after a week and broke up with him giving an excuse that he was not her type. To date, Sam did not know the reason why she dumped him. Georgina enrolled herself for the architect course but half-way realized she was not interested, so she discontinued the course. She started learning piano as that seemed to fascinate her. This went on with multiple courses and her mind kept wandering. A home was the most dreadful place for Georgina. Georgina would usually stay up at her friend's place or at one of her boyfriend's place. She always needed somebody to be around her all the time. Although she had a couple of very close friends who would advise her to be more affirmative and decisive. But all the advices would only stick to her mind for a short period and then it would be back to her routine.

Georgina took up a job with the Subway, as she was never able to complete any of the professional courses she took. One of the reasons for taking up the job was that all her friends were working somewhere, so she also wanted to work and keep herself busy. Her father would regularly send her money, so she never needed to work. She met Holmes who was a school dropout at her work. Holmes was a very confident person and was always quick to make any decision. He was very confident in spite of not having any higher education. He would tell Georgina that studies only make you learn but the ability to think comes when you believe yourself. They started enjoying each other's company and would spend a lot of time together. As Georgina's father was out most of the time, Holmes shifted to her place. This was the longest relationship she had ever had. She would occasionally date other boys, when Holmes was busy. Although Holmes knew about it he wouldn't mind it as he knew about Georgina's problem. He didn't believe in forcing a relationship on anyone. Holmes believed that with time Georgina would get over it. Holmes would encourage Georgina to overcome her indecisiveness. Her habit of self-doubting her decisions was one of the things which had always bothered Georgina. She had taken many courses for improving her self-confidence but most of them had a temporary effect. Even the Subway job which she had taken, she got bored out of it and as advised by her friends, she decided to quit it after a year. She would easily get influenced by people and if someone would create a doubt she would panic and rethink about the merits and demerits. Holmes was the perfect match for her temperament. He would be very calm with her and would help her overcome the panic and make the right decisions. Georgina would ask Holmes to give direct advice about what her mother did rather than talking around the bush. Holmes, on the other hand, would refrain from giving her solutions rather would assist her to solve problems. They were a perfect couple. Holmes had proposed Georgina a couple of times to marry her, but she would always refuse to say that she was not ready. Holmes would give her time to come up with the right decision and did not want to force her. Georgina meanwhile started working in a beauty parlour and was doing reasonably well. She seemed to have settled down with a permanent job and had a liking for it. This gave Holmes hopes that someday they could marry and start a family. She would spend maximum time with Holmes and her extra dates slowly started vanishing. She appreciated Holmes attitude of giving her space to think and felt she was lucky to have him.

Once when her supervisor was on a leave and Georgina was alone in the parlour. Since it was a Christmas Eve, there wasn't so much of a crowd in the street. A group of gangsters entered the parlour and stole the money at the gunpoint. Georgina was very scared. She had felt the guns' nozzle against her forehead as the gangsters threatened her to give them the keys of the cash vault. She quietly listened to the gangster fearing for her life. Once they disappeared with loot, she tried to call up Holmes. His phone was not reachable as the battery was dead. She frantically called him as she didn't know what to do, but he was not answering her phone. The gangster had warned her not to call up the cops, or they would come after her. Georgina was scared and confused what to do next. Should she call up her supervisor who was on a leave? Scared and shocked she cuddled herself next to the cashiers table. After 4 hours when an old customer came she saw Georgina scared and crying. She asked her what was the matter and Georgina told her that parlour had been robbed. The supervisor's number was written just next to the place where Georgina was sitting. It was the customer who called up the supervisor. The supervisor in turn called up the cops. Georgina who was shaken up was dropped at her home by the cops. When Holmes reached home, he was shocked to find Georgina in a miserable state. She told him the whole incident and asked him why he didn't pick up the phone. She blamed him that if his phone had been working, things would not have been so miserable. The gangsters would have been caught if he had alerted the cops. Only if he had picked up her phone. Holmes was puzzled at the bizarre logic but didn't want to upset Georgina. The CCTV footage was recovered and the gangsters were identified threatening Georgina. The CCTV footage also showed how Georgina was frantically calling up someone, and then she simply sat down doing nothing but crying. When the owner saw the video footage, she was perplexed with her behaviour. She realized that Georgina could not fit to handle stressful situation. She decided to fire her for her behaviour as she needed someone more responsible and upright. It was a small parlour, and she needed more responsible employees. The whole parlour was left unattended and Georgina was not even able to call and inform the management. This sounded extreme and unfair to Georgina who was already fighting her fears. She in turn blamed Holmes for not picking up the phone. One of her friends joked with her that if Holmes could not be with her in times of crisis what the point in having him in her life. She wasn't serious but just to make the situation lighter she had said this. Georgina got serious and started doubting her relationship with Holmes. She felt Holmes was avoiding her. This would lead to a lot of fights between them and finally, she broke up with Holmes. So, once again Georgina was alone in her life. She joined another Parlour which was in the Market area. All this had drained Georgina because of the broken relationship with the parlour incident first and now Homes out of her life. Holmes was tired of her tantrums and decided to move on. He had met another girl Alice in his workplace and decided to settle with her. He wanted to forget Georgina. Alice was always attracted to Holmes from first day of her job. Holmes and Alice got married just after a couple months of Georgina's breakup. Georgina meanwhile tried to divert her mind into work. She had taken up a job with a much lesser pay as she wanted to keep herself busy. She occasionally dated a few guys she knew, but she was not able to forget Holmes. Georgina missed his caring and understanding nature which had become a part of her life. Georgina was lonely and tried to end her life a couple of times. But she simply couldn't gather the courage. She realized she had been unfair to Holmes and decided to apologize to him. She went to his house after 6 months of her break up. Georgina was surprised to see Alice opening the door. Holmes came on the door and saw Georgina. Her face showed it all. She was guilty. Alice told her that they were married. Hearing this Georgina was shattered. First her Mom and now Holmes. Life had been very unfair with her. Alice decided to leave

Holmes and Georgina alone. Alice was a very soft girl and she trusted Holmes. Holmes made her sit on the sofa and told her to calm down. He explained to her that he had realized he couldn't stay with her post their break up. Alice just entered the room with some coffee. Alice told Georgina it wasn't her fault as Holmes told her about her past. Georgina was annoyed and she started cursing Alice. She called her a "housebreaker". Georgina stormed out of the house. Holmes told as she was leaving that her problems are not in her present but in her past. She needs to trust the right people and above all trust herself. Georgina was heartbroken. She realized she was all alone again. Deep in thoughts about her future Georgina reached home. It was dark and the lights were not working, she lit the candles, but she didn't realize that she had lit the candles very close to the curtains. The curtains caught fire. Slowly the furniture and the house was on fire. She realized it only when the whole house was burning, and she ran out of the house. The neighbours had already called the Fire brigade. All her savings, her belongings were doused in fire. Georgina knew she was in deep trouble, and she was homeless. All this was happening because of her fickle-mindedness. She was tired of her behaviour, and she wanted to get rid of it. She had lost her love, her job and now her house because of this dreadful cycle. Georgina went to the top a skyscraper to commit suicide, but she couldn't jump off. Frustrated and dejected she went to her friends place.

We are aware of the human's need for appreciation and rewards as discussed in previous chapters. The nucleus accumbens is responsible for dopamine to be released which in turns makes us happy. But there is another thing that humans crave for. We have learned in our school-days that humans like other mammals are social animals. Like we have other emotional and physical needs, the need for social interaction and its understanding is highly understated and overlooked. The learning for social interaction starts at an early age. The way the mother smiles at the new-born. How she cuddles him when he is crying, the child is silently learning social behaviours. Some scientists believe that the familiarity with the mother's voice is during the gestation period where the only sound he hears is the mother's voice. The brain is highly plastic in nature and all the neuronal circuits are formed in the new-born but not yet connected. We do inherit some fixed circuits at our births but the majority is governed by our experiences. This need for social interactions increases with time but the neuronal circuits formed by experience greatly influences our social interaction. The craving to be appreciated or loved is one of the prime reasons responsible for our interactions. To be a part of peer group starts from early childhood till we die. Those who adapt easily are highly popular and the ones who are not, get rejected. This does not decrease the craving and hence people behave in a way which they are not comfortable with. The Orbitofrontal cortex (OFC) is responsible for helping us to adapt to people from different ethnic religion and behaviours. It makes us more tolerant of diverse viewpoints and become emotionally intelligent. Being dependent on people is also one of the social behaviours which we adopt from early childhood because of overprotection by parents and family members. This makes us less self-confident creating conditions for decreased self-regulation and amygdala to fire leading to stress and anxiety. Peer pressure is one of the most common problems with teens and their desire to change themselves to be a part of the group is a prime stressor in their age group. Parents who make decisions for kids especially teen and do not give them the freedom to choose are actually crippling them to face the world in future as in the case of Georgina. The ability to differentiate between wrong and right is a highly complex brain function involving the prefrontal lobe and the parietal lobe. Pampering and being overprotective to safeguard the child leads to complex problems for them in later life. Getting awareness in spite of the efforts seemed to be futile for Georgina in later life. Holmes did try to help her, but he was not able to rewire her thought processes.

Insight

Every parent wants their children to have minimum sufferings in their life. They do not want them to go through the same struggles, which they have faced in their lives. However, some parents end up being overprotective. They start making decisions for them. Children, when they are in primary school, need to be protected. They should be given enough space so they can learn how to make the right decisions. This is often ignored by many parents until their teenage life. But when this over protectiveness of parents spills in adult life, it ends up damaging their self-confidence.

When parents criticize their children too much for the wrong decision they make, the children develop a fear for trying new things. This destroys their creativity and self-confidence.

Children become indecisive and become dependent on their family or friends for making decisions. This is more common in some conservative families. Striving the right balance between watchful monitoring and active decision-making is one of the biggest challenges, parents have to face when they deal with teenage children.

After her mother's death, Georgina found it difficult to deal with everyday challenges of life. Parents, when they are too dominating, create hassles for their children in adult life. This created self-doubt in Georgina who lost the ability to explore new challenges. The ability to analyse situations was lost. This spilled over to her relationship with other boys and her career. She ended up losing the interest in her career as no analysis was ever done before making a decision. Such people are very vulnerable to marketers and are easily exploited by people for their own benefit. When Georgina was caught into the

burglary episode she did not know how to manage
herself and expected Holmes to rescue her.

Georgina had to understand the root cause of her
problem and try to find the necessary solutions.
She needed to understand why she was so fickle
minded and how she could slowly start making
decisions without the fear of failing.

As Georgina was sitting at her friends place
wondering what to do next. She knew she had
goofed and was aware of her issue for a long
time. She wanted to get over her problem. Her
friend advised her to take a break and spend some
time at her villa in the countryside. Hesitant but
she had no choice. The villa was looked after by
an 82-year-old caretaker. Her friend used to spend
time at the villa whenever she wanted to take a
break. As Georgina was sitting in the villa staring
at the coast nearby. She felt a hand touching her
shoulder. It was the same lady. Georgina saw the
compassion in her eyes. The lady asked Georgina
what was the problem? Georgina did not want to
share her problem with a stranger, so she told she
was all right. She only wanted to take a break
from her life. She was too stressed about her
work. The old lady smiled and told her she was
always there whenever she needs to speak to
someone. It gets very lonely if you don't share
your sorrows and trouble. The old lady left the
room. Georgina tried to avoid looking at the lady
as she was scared she would read her pain if she

looked in her eyes. On the fourth day, there was a thunderstorm and was raining heavily. She was looking out of the window when the old lady came into the room. She told Georgina, "Nature is the biggest healer in the world. Get close to it and trust nature. To get wet in the rain is the best way to hide your tears". She left the room after saying this. Georgina was already thinking of getting wet. But she feared to catch a cold. Her head was already hurting after thinking so hard and getting wet in the rain seemed to be an interesting proposition. As she was drenched in the rain she felt calm. She started remembering Holmes and tears rolled down her cheeks. Georgina closed her eyes and trusted nature. Her head went numb and felt light. She came back into the villa. The old lady was at the door with a towel in her hand. Georgina wiped herself and thanked the lady. Georgina went to the old lady's room after she changed her clothes. The old lady greeted her. Georgina asked her who she was and how she came to know that there was some problem in her life. The old lady smiled. She told her that she was in this house for the last 50 years and when she met Georgina her eyes told her that she was in deep pain. Georgina wanted to share her problem. The old lady made her feel comfortable and told her that she does not need to tell her as she was not connected to the fast city life, which Georgina was living. She was a villager and had no idea about the complexities of her life. But she can share her woes if it would make her feel better. Georgina told her about her indecisiveness. How from early childhood she feared to make decisions? Her affair with Holmes and how things had turned out. She wept as she was telling her story to the old lady. The old smiled at her and told her that Georgina had suffered a lot in her life because of that. The only problem she felt was that Georgina wanted people to help her. The solution was in herself. Like she went and got wet she needs to find a solution and trust that she can find the best possible answer to her infinite problems. The old lady told her that she was a very brave lady, much stronger than her. But she needs to find her strength and the journey is lonely. Nobody can help her. Georgina felt puzzled by the answer. She expected some advice from her but the old lady was simply telling her to find an answer herself. Seeing the puzzled look on her face the old lady told her in her ears whatever you decide doesn't matter but what matters is that you are comfortable. Left confused as always, Georgina smiled and left the room. She couldn't forget the old lady's words. She recollected and started writing down all the major incidents of her life on the paper and their outcome. Then she wrote down all the possible outcomes which she wanted. As she was writing down she also realized that the things could have gone wrong if she chose option B, and she would be having the same pain. Then what difference would it make if she had opted for option A or B. What mattered was that she needed to be comfortable with her decisions. Life was not about making perfect decisions but to live the imperfect ones and making them work. She understood what the old lady wanted to tell her.

She realized the problem was never why she made a decision but how much she believed in it. With renewed energy, she decided to go back to work next morning. She thanked the old lady and left. She went to the insurance office as she had a fire insurance for the house. She rented a place for a few days with the savings in the bank. Georgina decided to sell the plot and took up a small place for opening her boutique. She decided to work independently and had directly approached her clientele with whom she had built a relationship in all these years. Her business picked up as she was very well tuned with her work. She bought the same plot and build her house again. She decided to meet Holmes and Alice and apologize for her behaviour. It so happened that Alice and Holmes had separated. Holmes wanted to reconcile with Georgina. Georgina told him that she had moved on but always respected him as a close friend. Holmes knew Georgina was a changed lady. He respected her decision. Georgina went to meet her friend whose villa she had been to. She had spoken to her on phone but wanted to know about the lady in her villa whom she had met a year back. Her friend informed Georgina that the lady had passed away. She had lost her husband and her son in an accident when she was just 30 years. Ever since she had been living alone in that house. People of her village had thrown her out considering her to be a bad omen and that's when her father had found her. She was the caretaker but her friend had never seen her sad or upset in her entire life. Georgina smiled as she remembered the old lady's words that "nature is the biggest healer in the world".

11.

Sam's Party

As the date started approaching, Sam was excited to meet all his old friends. It was as if, he was traveling back in time. He wanted this to be the most memorable event, as he would introduce Jane and Anna to his past. He had booked a big hall on the seventh floor where all the guest could be easily accommodated. There were Sam and Jane's relatives and office colleagues also but Sam was very much keen on seeing his old mates. He had bought for himself a brand-new Armani suit. Jane and Anna could see the excitement on his face, and they too wanted to meet Sam's friends. Sam had arranged for live music and told the whole room to be decorated with candles. Although initially, the management had refused giving safety reasons. Sam and his manipulative ways of talking convinced them finally. He had called all Anna's friend and arranged a different room on the same floor, where the youngster could enjoy themselves. Anna was really grateful to her father for trusting her and her friends. He gave them the space to enjoy the party alone. She was happy to see the changes in her father.

As the guest started arriving, Sam like a good host was at the door, receiving them. A hand from the back tapped on his head. He turned behind to see, Tom and George standing behind him. He didn't recognize them at first but when they told them who they were, Sam was really excited to see them. They had come with their family and children. Slowly all the guests started arriving. He

had arranged a separate corner for his old mates
and their family. All his friends arrived except
Kim. Sam welcomed everyone and started talking
about his journey with everyone. How he rescued
his daughter and learned from his mistakes. Sam
was very happy and he hugged his daughter and
wife, to thank them to be a part of his wonderful
journey of life. As he was talking he saw a lady in
a wheelchair entering the room. He went to the
door and welcomed her. He was surprised to
know that it was Kim, and she had lost her legs in
an accident.

All the ten mates with their families were having
a good time. They were reliving their past and
were cracking jokes with each other. Times had
changed but the child in them was alive on that
day. They were all sharing their lives without the
fear of being judged or analysed. Each one had a
story to tell. As they narrated their stories they
realized what seemed like a simple journey in
their childhood days was very complicated and
full of hardships. As the friends were listening
intently to what all had happened in their lives,
they realized that there is a story waiting to be
told. Which is unique and difficult in itself. They
were happy that they could all meet up finally.
Sharing their journey gave them the insight which
each of them would add the gain to their character
in some form. Sam who initially thought that his
life had a lot of ups and downs realized that there
were Kim and Georgina who had faced a lot more
and were living examples of courage.

Moses,Frank,Thomas,Tom,Lucy,Georgina,Dr.Ge
orge,Kim and Hemant forgot their sorrows and

realised challenges were in everybody's life. They all felt a sense of pride to have batch mates who were so brave and never gave up. The room was full of positive energy. They did not bow down to the hardships and challenges, life gave them and fought with vigour and courage. As the crowd started leaving, ten of them sat down alone to till late evening. They didn't realize where time was flying away.

Sam went into another room where Anna and the other kids were dancing to music. He saw his friend's kids getting along well in spite of them meeting for the first time. Sam was surprised and called the other friends to see how they were getting along so well. Tom said in a lighter vein that they had inherited these relationships. It was very refreshing for everyone to see the kids playing along. It reminded them of the good old days. Life was way too simple even though the fixed or hardwired neuronal circuits which were formed in their minds were not causing any trouble. They realized life had become way too complicated for them as they grew up but deep down their heart and mind they were still thinking and feeling like those kids playing around. They had all learned a lot about their shortcomings and at times complicated thinking through various life experiences. These laws of neuroplasticity were applicable to each and every individual at different phases of their life but the actual need arose as life got complicated. They were thankful that they had gotten over those dreadful lessons from life and had rewired as we all do with our experiences. Frank told that they hope they do not have to read and experience the laws of neuroplasticity ever in their lives. All the friends smiled as they looked at each other at Frank's statements. They knew life would be throwing a challenge again and these laws will come to their rescue. Life was never predictable and will never be for anyone. It's these laws which keep reminding us that life is beautiful, provided we change with changing times.

12.

Looking beyond the horizon.

One most common things about the laws and the book is that, they are deep-rooted to the connections with the childhood events. Interventions did in the early childhood, especially with relevance of expanding the horizon of awareness. It will help in applying it to various aspects of the child's behaviour and understanding of human emotions will reap rich benefits. This would, in turn, avoid getting them entangled in the webs of fixed thinking and rigid thoughts.

These laws lay down the foundation for reaping the positive gains at a later stage in the child's life. Interventions at an adult stage with people having fixed and rigid thinking have much lesser impact as compared to the young children. As the advances in technology seems to be the order of the day, the lack of awareness and automation in the brain circuit also seems to be diminishing at a rapid rate. Just a simple glance around you in a public place, will prove, the speed with the human brain seems to be in automation and dependent on technology. Training of children at a young age along with academics in the science of awareness and socio-emotional aspect, seems to be the most prudent and long-lasting solution to the future generation we can give.

References

1. 1913 classic: Watson, J.B. 1913. Psychology as the behaviorist views. Psychological Review, 20 pp. 158-177. Exposure and response prevention: Baer, L., & Minichello, W. E.1998.
2. Behavioral treatment for OCD. In: Jenike, M.A., Baer, L., & Minichiello, W. E. [Eds.] 1998. Obsessive-compulsive disorders: Practical management, 3rd ed. St. Louis: Mosby scientism: Barzun, J. 2000. From dawn to decadence: 500 years of Western cultural life. New York: HarperCollins, p. 218.
3. Bare Attention: Nyanaponika Thera. 1973. The heart of Buddhist meditation. York Beach, Maine: Samuel Weiser, p. 30.
4. Impartial and well-informed spectator: Smith, A, 1976. Raphael. D., & Macfie, A. L., [Eds.] the theory of moral sentiments. New York: Oxford University Press, pp. 112-113.
5. "The essential achievement of the will". James, W. 1983. The principles of psychology. Cambridge, Mass.: Harvard University Press, p.1166.

"Prolong the stay in consciousness":
Ibid. p. 429.
"The utmost a believer in free-will can
ever do": Ibid. p. 1177.
"Choose and sculpt how our ever-
changing minds": Merzenich, M. M., &
deCharms, R. 1996.
Neural representations, experience, and
change. In: Llinas, R., & Church land,
P.S. [Eds.] the mind-Brain continuum:
Sensory processes. Cambridge, Mass:
MIT Press, pp. 62-81.

6. "User illusion": Dennett, D. 1994. In:
    Guttenplan, S. A companion to the
    philosophy of mind. Oxford, U. K:
    Blackwell, pp. 236-243.

7. Alcmaeon of Croton: Burnet, J. 1920.
    Early Greek philosophy, 3rded. London:
    A & C. Black.

8. ''the brain has the most power for man":
    Hippocrates, on the sacred disease.
    Translation from Kirk, G.S., & Raven,
    J.E.1963.The pre-Socratic philosophers:
    A critical history with a selection of
    texts. New York: Cambridge University
    Press, p.442.

9. Stimulated tiny spots on the surface:
    Penfield, W., &Perot, P. 1963.

10. The brain's record of auditory and visual
    experience. Brain, 86, Pp., 595-697.

11. "The word Mind is obsolete'': Bogen, J.
    E.1998. My developing Understanding
    of Roger Wolcott Sperry's philosophy.

Neuropsychologia, 36 (10), pp.1089-1096.

12. "Understand the brain'': Nichols, M.J...& Newsome, W.T. 1999.The Neurobiology of cognition. Nature, 402, p. C35-38.

13. "The fundamental features of [the physical] world are as described by physics": Searle, J.R.200. A philosopher unriddles the puzzle of Consciousness. Cerebrum, 2, pp. 44-54.

14. Explanatory gap: Levine, J. 1983. Materialism and qualia: The Explanatory gap. Pacific Philosophical Quarterly, 6, pp. 354-361.

15. Imagine a conscious minds in a material world. New York: Basic Books, p. 28.

16. "That one body may act upon another''. The Correspondence of Isaac Newton. Volume III, 1688-1694. Edited by H. W. Turnbull,

17. F.R.S. Cambridge: Published for the Royal Society at the University Press, 1961. Letter 406 Newton to Bentley, 25 February 1692/3.

18. One version of quantum theory: Von Neumann. J. 1932. Mathema-Tische Grundlagen der Quanten Mechanik. English translation from Beyer, R.T.1953. Mathematical foundations of quantum mechanics.Princeton, N. J: Princeton University Press.

19. Descartes and La Metrie: see the discussion of their work in: Reck, A.J. 1972. Speculative philosophy: A study of its nature, types, and Uses. Albuquerque: University of New Mexico Press.

20. As Colin McGinn puts it: McGinn, 1999, pp. 18-19.

21. Steven Rose: Rose, S. 1998. Brains, mind and the world. In: Rose, S. (Ed.).

22. From brain to consciousness: Essays on the new sciences of the   mind. Princeton, N.J.: Princeton   University Press, p.12.

23. "That our being should consist of two fundamental elements": Sherrington, C. S. 1947 .The integrative action of the nervous system, 2d Ed. New Haven, Conn.: Yale University Press, p. Xxxiv.

24. In   1986   Eccles proposed: Eccles, J. C.1986.Do mental events cause neural events analogously to the probability fields of quantum mechanics? Proceedings of the Royal Society of London. Series B: Biological Sciences, 227, pp. . . . . 411 – 428.

25. Among the warring theories: Edelman, G. M., & Tononi, G .A. 2000.

26. Universe of consciousness: How matter becomes imagination. New York: Basic Books, p. 6.

27. "Mentalistic Materialism": as the neurosurgeon Joe Bogen has termed it: Bogen, 1998.

28. "Mental processes are just brain processes": Flanagan. 1992.

29. Consciousness reconsidered. Cambridge, Mass; MIT Press, p. Xi...Church land and Daniel Dennett: Church land, P.M., & Church land, P.S.1998 .On the contrary: Critical   essays, 1987-1997. Cambridge,

30. Mass: MIT Press: Dennett, D.C.1991. Consciousness explained. Boston: Little, Brown.

31. "Mind does not move matter": Herrick, C. J. 1956. The evolution of human nature. Austin, Tex.: University of Texas Press, p. 281.

32. The causal efficacy of mind: James, W. 1983. The automaton theory.

33. In: The principles of psychology. Cambridge Mass: Harvard University Press, Chap. 5.Called such trains spandrels: Gould, S. J., & Lewontin, R. C. 1979.

34. The spandrels of San Marco and the Panglossian paradigm: a critique of the adaptationist program. Proceedings of the Royal Society of London B, 205, pp. 581-598.

35. Emerging materialism: Sperry, R. W. 1992. Turnabout on consciousness: A mentalist view. Journal of Mind and Behavior, 13, pp. 259-280.

36. As he put it in 1970: Sperry. R.W. 1970.
    Perception in the absence of the
    neocortical commissures. Research
    Publications Association for Research in
    Nervous and Mental Disease, 48, pp.
    123-138.
37. Agnostic physicalism: Bogen, 1998.
38. Process philosophy: for a useful
    overview see Reck, A. J. 1972... A useful
    book on Whitehead's profoundly
    abstract philosophical system is
    Sherburn, D. W. [Ed.] 1981. A key to
    Whitehead's process and reality.
    Chicago: University of Chicago Press.
39. Dualistic interactionism: Popper, K. R.,
    & Eccles J. C> 1977. The self and its
    brain: An argument for interactionism.
    New York: Springer International. The
    Australian philosopher David Chalmers:
    Chalmers, D. J. 1996.
40. The conscious mind: In search of a
    fundamental theory. New York: Oxford
    University Press.
    "Started out life as a materialist": Kuhn,
    R. L. 2000. Closer to the truth. New
    York: McGraw-Hill, P. 21.
41. "To truly bridge the gap". Ibid.
42. "When I first got interested in": Searle,
    2000
43. Crick: Crick, F.J. 1994. The astonishing
    hypothesis: The scientific search for the
    soul. New York: Scribner's.
44. Edelman: Edelman & Tononi, 2000.

"Reductionist neurobiological
explanations": Singer, W. 1998.

45. Consciousness from a neurobiological
perspective. In: Rose [Ed.] 1998, p. 229.
"Ambiguous relationship to mind".
Rose, 1998.
"Mind is but the babbling of a robot".
Doty, R. W. 1998. The five mysteries of
the mind, and their consequences.
Neuropsychologia, 36, pp. 1069-1076.

46. Obsessive compulsive disorder [OCD]:
Two standard reference books for
information on OCD are: Jenike, M. A.,
Baer, L., & Minichieo, W. E. [Eds.]
1998. Obsessive-compulsive disorders:
Practical management, 3rd ed. St. Louis:
Mosby, Koran,

47. L. M. 1999. Obsessive- compulsive and
related disorders in adults: A
comprehensive clinical guide. New
York: Cambridge University Press.

48. Exposure and response prevention: Foe,
E. B., & Wilson, R. 2001.

49. Stop obsessing! How to overcome your
obsessions and compulsions, rev. Ed.
New York: Bantam Doubleday Del;
Meyer V., Levy, R., & Schnurer, A.
1974.
The behavioral treatment of obsessive-
compulsive disorders In: Beech, H. R.
[Ed.] Obsessional states. London:
Methuen, pp. 233-256.
Some 25 percent of patients: Baer, L., &
Minichello, W. E. 1998.

50. Behavioral treatment for obsessive-compulsive disorder. In: Jenike, Baer, & Minichiello, 1998, pp. 337-367.

51. Cognitive therapy---a form of structured introspection---was already widely used: Back, A. T., Rush, A. J., Shaw, B. F., & Emery, G, 1979.

52. Cognitive therapy of depression, New York: Guilford Press.

53. We had studied depression: Baxter, L. R., Jr., M.E., MazzIotta, J. C., Schwartz, J. M., et al. 1985. Cerebral metabolic rates for Glucose in mood disorders: Studies with positron emission tomography and fluorodeoxyglucose F 18. Archives of General Psychiatry, 42, pp. 441-447.

54. Analysis of the PET scans: Baxter, L, R., Jr., Schwartz, J. M., Mazziotta, J C., et al .1988.

55. Cerebral glucose metabolic rates in non-depressed patients with obsessive – compulsive disorder. American Journal of Psychiatry, 145, pp. 1560-1563; Baxter, L.R., Jr., Phelps, M .E., Mazziotta, J. C., Guze, B. H., Schwartz, J. M., & Selin, C.E.1987.

56. Local cerebral glucose metabolic   rates in obsessive-compulsive Disorder: A comparison with rates in unipolar depressive and in normal controls. Archives of General Psychiatry, 44, PP.211-128.

57. Anterior cingulated gyros: Swedo, S. E., Schapiro, M.B., Grady, C. L., et al. 1989. Cerebral glucose metabolism in childhood-onset obsessive-compulsive disorder. Archives of General Psychiatry, 46, pp. 518-523.

58. Elevated metabolism in the orbital frontal cortex: Rauch, S. L., & Baxter, L.R. 1998. Neuroimaging in obsessive-compulsive disorder and related disorders. In: Jenike, Baer, & Minichiello, 1998, pp. 289-317.

59. Behavioral physiologist E. T. Rolls at Oxford : Thorpe, S. J., Rolls,

60. E.T., & Madison's. 1983. The orbitofrontal cortex: Neuronal activity in the behaving monkey. E experimental Brain Research, 4, pp. . . . . 93- 115.

61. The orbital frontal cortex, it seems, functions as an error detector:

62. Reviews of recent work on this subject are in: Rolls, E. T. 2000. The Orbitofrontal cortex and reward. Cerebral Cortex, 10,pp.284 – 294;

63. O'Doherty, J., Kringbach, M.., Rolls, E. T., et al. 2001. Abstract reward and punishment representations in the human orbitofrontal cortex. Nature Neuroscience, 4, pp. . . .95 -102; Rogers R. D., Owen,

64. A.M., Middleton, H .C. et al. 1999.Choosing between small, likely rewards and large, unlikely rewards activates inferior and orbital prefrontal

cortex. Journal of Neuroscience, 15, pp. 9029-9038.

65. Volunteers pay a sort of gambling game: Bechara, A., Damasio, H., Tranel, D., & Damasio, A. R. 1997. Deciding Advantageously before knowing the advantageous strategy. Science, 275, pp. 1293 -1295.
Bechara, A., Damasio, H., Damasio, A.R., & Lee, G. P. 1999. Different contributions of the human amygdala and ventromedial prefrontal cortex to decision –making. Journal of Neuroscience, 19, pp. . . . . 5473-5481.

66. Traffic pattern connecting the striatum and the cortex: For accessible reviews of this see: Schwartz, J. M., 1998. Neuroanatomical aspects of cognitive-behavioral therapy response in obsessive- compulsive disorder: An evolving perspective on brain and behavior. British Journal of Psychiatry, 173, Supplement 35, pp. 39-45; Schwartz, J. M. 1997.

67. Obsessive –compulsive disorder. Science & Medicine, 4 (2), pp.14-23.are called matrices: Eblen, F., & Graybiel, A.M. 1995. Highly restricted origin of prefrontal cortical inputs to striosomes in the macaque monkey. Journal of Neuroscience, 15, pp.599 -6013neuronal mosaic of reason and passion: Graybiel, A. M., & Rauch, S.L.2000. Toward a

neurobiology of obsessive –compulsive disorder. Neuron,28, pp. 343 – 347;

68.   Graybiel, A. M. & Canales, J.J. 2001. The neurobiology of repetitive behaviors; clues to the neurobiology of Tourette syndrome. Advances in Neurology, 85, pp. 123 -131. Topically active neurons (TANs): Osaka, T., Kimura, M., & Graybiel, A.M.1995. Temporal and spatial characteristic of tonic ally active neurons of the primate's striatum. .Journal of Neurophysiology, 73, 1234 -1252.

69. Serve as sort of gating mechanism, redirecting information flow: Graybiel, A. M. 1998. The basal ganglia and chunking of action and Repertoires. Neurobiology of Learning and Memory, 70, pp. 119-136.

70. Role in the development of Habits: Jog, M. S., Kubota, Y., and Connolly. I., Hildegard, V., & Graybiel, A. M. 1999. Building neural representations of habits. Science, 26, pp. 1745-1749.

71. Purposefully alter the response contingencies of their own TANs: Schwartz, J.M. 1999. A role for volition and attention in the generation of new brain circuitry: Toward a neurobiology of mental force.

72. In: Liber, B., Freeman, A., & Sutherland, K. [Eds.]. The volitional Brain: Towards a neuroscience of free will. Thorvertion, U. K.: Imprint Academic.

73. Two output pathway: one direct and one indirect: Baxter, L. R., Jr., Clark, E. C., Iqbal, M., & Ackermann, R. F. 2001. Cortical-subcortical Systems in the mediation of obsessive-compulsive disorder: Modeling the brain's mediation of a classic "neurosis, "In: Lichter, D. G., & Cummings, J. L. [Eds.] Frontal-subcortical circuits in psychiatric and neurological disorders. New York: Guilford Press, pp. 207-230. "Worry circuit": Baxter, L. R., Jr. Schwartz, J. M., et al. 1992. Caudate glucose metabolic rate changes with both drug and behavior Therapy for obsessive-compulsive disorder. Archives of General Psychiatry, 43, pp. 681-689.

74. "Streams of thought and motivation". Graybiel & Rauch, 2000.

75. What I came to call Brain Lock: Schwartz, J. M., * Beyette, B. 1997.

76. Brain lock: Free yourself from obsessive-compulsive behavior. New York: HarperCollins.

77. Anterior cingulated: Bush, G., Lou, P., & Posner, M. I. 2000. Cognitive and emotional influences in anterior cingulated cortex. Trends in Cognitive Sciences, 4, pp. 215-222.

78. Researchers at Massachusetts General Hospital: Breiter, H. C., Rauch, S. L., et al. 1996. Functional magnetic resonance imaging of Symptom provocation in obsessive-

compulsive disorder. Archives of
General Psychiatry, 53, pp. 595-606;
Rauch, S. L., Jenike, M. A., et
al. 1994. Regional cerebral blood flow
measured during symptom
Provocation in obsessive-compulsive
disorder using oxygen

79. 15-labeled carbon dioxide and positron
emission tomography.
Archives of General Psychiatry, 51, pp.
62-70.
Nyanaponika Thera: Nyanaponika thera,
1973.

80. Ludwig von Miss, who defined valuing:
Von Misses, L. 1962. The ultimate
foundation of economic science: An
essay on method.

81. Kansas City, Kans: Shed Andrews &
Mamet.
Significantly diminished metabolic
activity: Schwartz, J. M., Stoes-sel, P.
W., Baxter, L. R., Jr., et al. 1996.
Systematic changes in cerebral glucose
metabolic rate after successful behavior
modification treatment of obsessive-
compulsive disorder. Archives of
General Psychiatry, 53, pp. 109-113.

82. Benison of Wayne State: Benazon, N.
R., Ager, J., & Rosenberg,
D. R. 2002. Cognitive behavior therapy
in treatment-naive children and
adolescents with obsessive-compulsive

disorder: An open trial.Behavior
Research and Therapy, 40, p. 529-539.

83. William James posed the question:
Meyers, G. E. [Ed.] 1992. Psychology:
Briefer course. In: William James
Writing's 1878-1899.New York: Library
of America. 417.

84. Lasting language deficit: Ratey, J. J.
2000. A user's guide to the brain.
New York: Pantheon, p.270.

85. To process visual information instead:
Eliot, Lise, 1999. What's going on in
there? How the brain and mind develop
in the first five years of life, New York:
Bantam, p. 250.

86. Congenitally deaf people: Bavelier, D.,
& Neville, H. J. 2002. Cross, Modal
plasticity: where and how? Nature
Reviews Neuroscience, 3 [6], pp. 443-
452.

87. In their breakthrough experiment: Von
Melchner, L., Pallas, S. L.,Sur, M. 2000
Visual behavior mediated by retinal
projections

88. Directed to the auditory pathway.
Nature, 404, pp. 871-875.
"The animals 'see'": Merzenenich, M.
2000. Seeing in the sound zone Nature,
404, pp. 820-821.

89. As a cause of behavioral improvements:
Van Praag, H., Kemper Mann, G., &
Gage, F. H. 2000. Neural consequences
of environmental enrichment. Nature
Reviews Neuroscience, 1, pp. 191-198.

90. Strengthened their synaptic connection:
    Robertson, I. H., & Murre, J. M. J. 1999.
    Rehabilitation of brain damage: Brain
    plasticity and principles of guided
    recovery. Psychological Bulletin, 125.pp.
    544-575.
    Molecular changes: Kandel, E R. 1998.
    A new intellectual framework for
    psychiatry. American Journal of
    Psychiatry, 155[4], pp. 457-469.
    An average of 2,500 of these specialized
    junctions, synapses: Gopnik, A.,
    Meltzoff, and A. N., & Kuhn, P.K.
    1999.The scientist in the crib:
91. Minds, brains and how children learn.
    New York: William Morrow,
    p. 186.
92. 100 trillion---synapses: Ibid. p. 181.
93. About half the neurons that form in the
    fetal brain die before the
    Baby is born: Ratey, 2000, p. 26.
    1.8 million Synapses per second: Eliot,
    1999, p. 27.
    20 billion synapses are pruned every
    day: Ibid. p. 32.
    They literally could not hear any
    difference: Gopnik, Meltzoff &
    Kuhn, 1999, p. 103.
    By twelve months they could not: Ibid.
    p. 107.
    Rarely learn to speak it like a native:
    Ibid. p. 192.

Forms millions of connections every day: Ibid. p. 1.

In the wild of New York City: Ibid. p. 182.

94. All of the 100 million neurons of the primary visual cortex form: Eliot, 199, p. 204.

10   Billion per day: Ibid.

11   Visual acuity has improved fivefold: Maurer, D., Lewis, T.L., Brent, H.P., & Levin, A. V. 1999. Rapid improvement in the acuity of Infants after visual input. Science, 286, pp.108-109.

12   See the world almost as well as well a normal adult: Sireteanu, R. 199.

13   Switching on the infant brain. Science, 286, pp. 58 – 59.

14   "Eliminate addressing errors'': Shatz C. J.1992. The developing brain Scientific American, 267, pp. 62 -67.

Strikes about 1 baby in 10,000: Sireteanu, 1999, p.60.

The brain never   develops the ability to see normally: Ibid. p.59.

"Visual input was focused on the retina": Maurer, 1999, p.108.

As well as normal language development: Sireteanu, 1999, p.61. Led by Elizabeth Sowell: Sowell, E. R., Thompson, P. M., Holmes,

15   C.J., Jernigan, T. L., Toga, A.W.
     199. In vivo evidence for post-
     Adolescent brain maturation in
     frontal and striatal regions. Nature
     Neuroscience, 2, pp.859 -861.

16   Increased through age eleven or
     twelve: Giedd, J .N. Blumenthal, J.,
     Jeffries N. O., Castellanos, F. X.,
     Liu, H., Zijdenbos, A., Paus, T.,
     Evans, A.C., Rapoport, J. L.
     1999.Brain development during
     childhood and adolescence: a
     longitudinal MRI study. Nature
     Neuroscience 2, pp.861 -863.

17   "In adult centers": In Lowenstein,
     D.H. & Parent, J. M.1999.Brian heal
     thyself. Science, 283, pp. 1126 -
     1127.

18   "We are still taught": Ibid p. 1126.
AS a student at Ohio State: Guillermo,
K.S.1983. Monkey business: The
disturbing case that launched the animal
rights movement. Washington, D. C.:
National Press Books, p. 32.
Bought at a toy store: Guillermo,
1983, p. 25.

19   The saga of the Silver Spring
     monkeys: for an excellent and
     concise
Account of the case, see Fraser,
Caroline. 1993. The raid at silver
Spring. The New Yorker, 69, p. 66.

20   In 1895 Sherrington: Reprinted in
     Denny—Brown, D. [Ed.] 1940.

Selected writings of Sir Charles
Sherrington. New York: Harper & Bros.
Pp. 115---119.
Reflecting on the 1895 results:
Sherrington, C.S. 1931. Hugh lings
21   Jackson Lecture. Brain, 54, pp. 1-28.
By 1947: Sherrington, 1947, pp. Xxi-
xxiii.
22   "A negative reinforce": Skinner,
     B.F. 1974. About Behaviorism. New
     York: Alfred A. Knopf, p.47.
23   Electric shock that lasted up to 3.5
     seconds: Taub, E. 1980.
Somatosensory deafferentation research
with monkeys: Implications for
rehabilitation medicine. In Inca, L. P.
[Ed.] Behavioral
24   Psychology in rehabilitation
     medicine. Baltimore: Williams
     &Wilkins, pp. 371-401.
25   "Was to be of long duration, if
     necessary'': Ibid. p. 374.
The monkey uses it: Taube, E. 1977.
Movement in nonhuman primates
deprived of somatosensory feedback.
Exercise and Sports Sciences   Reviews,
4, pp. 335-374.
26   "Except   the most precise": Ibid.
     p.368.
"Potentially useful": Ibid. p. 342.
"Major difficulties in carrying out
deafferentation experiments with
monkeys": Ibid. p.343.

Six out of eleven fetuses died: Ibid.
p.359.
"Are not the inevitable consequences of
deafferentation'': Guillermo, 1983,
p.133.
"Let the monkeys go?" Kilpatrick, J.
1986. Jailed in Poolesville. The
Washington Post, May 12, A 15.
The fifteen surviving monkeys: Dajer, T.
1992. Monkeying with the brain.
Discover, 13, p. 70.
27   "Had been through hell and back":
     Ibid.
When they were three or four years old:
Pons, T. P., Garreaghty, P. E., ommaya,
A. K., Kaas, J. H., Taub, E., & Mishkin,
M. 1991. Massive cortical reorganization
after sensory deafferentation in adult
Macaques, Science, 252, pp. 1857-1860.
"A couple of millimeters": Ibid. p. 1857.
28   Paul stopped eating: Goldstein, A.
     A. 1990. Silver Spring monkey
Undergoes final experiment. The
Washington Post, January 22,
E 3
Rejected the advice: Dajer, 1992.
Help up experiments on the seven
surviving monkeys: Barnard,
N. D. 1990. Animal experimentation:
The case of the Silver Spring
Monkeys. The Washington Post,
February 25, B 3.

"Euthanized for humane reasons":
Sullivan, L. W. 1990. Free for all:
Morality and the monkeys. The
Washington Post, March 17, a 27.was
denied on April 12, 1991: Okie, S. S., &
Jennings, V. 1991. Rescued animals
killed: Animal rights group defends
euthanasia. The Washington Post, April
13, A 1.he never awoke: Ibid.
29 "Advantageous to study the Silver
     Spring monkey": Supple, C. 1991.
Brain's ability to rewire after injury is
extensive; "Silver Spring monkeys" used
in research. The Washington Post. June
28, A 3. "A distinct and different
essence": Penfield, W. 1975.
30 The mystery of the mind. Princeton,
     N. J.: Princeton University Press, p.
     55, 62.chapter on habit: James,
     1983, p. 110.
31 In 1912 T. Graham Brown and
     Charles Sherrington: Graham
     Brown, T., & Sherrington, C. S.
     1912. On the instability of a cortical
     Point. Proceedings of Royal Science
     Society of London, 85 B, pp. 250-
     277.
32 S. lvory Franz compared movement
     map: Franz, S. I. 1915. Variations in
     distribution of the motor centers.
     Psychological Review, Monograph
     Supplement 19, pp. 80-162.

33   Sherrington himself described "the
     excitable cortex": Layton, A.F.S., &
     Sherrington, C. S. 1917.
     Observations on the excitable cortex
     of the chimpanzee, orangutan and
     goria. Quarterly Journal
Of Experimental Physiology, 1, pp. 135-
222.
34   Karl Lashley, a former colleague of
     Franz: Lashley, K. S. 1923.
     Temporal variation in the function
     of the guru's precentralis in
     primates.
35   American Journal of Physiology 65,
     pp. 585-602.
"Plasticity of neural function": Lashley,
K. S. 1926.
Neurology 4, pp. 1-58
Remodeled continually by experience:
Merzenich, M. M., & Jenkins. M. 1993.
Cortical representations of learned
behaviors. In: Andersen, P. et al. [Ed.]
Memory concepts. New York: Elsevier,
pp.437-454.
36   Donald Hebb postulated coincident-
     based synaptic plasticity:
Hebb, D. O. 1949. The organization of
behavior: A neuropsychological theory.
New York: John Wiley.
37   The great Spanish neuroanatomist
     Ramon y Cajal: DeFelipe, J.,
     &Jones, E. G. [Eds.] 1988. Ramon y
     Cajal Santiago: Cajal on the cerebral

cortex: An annotated translation of the complete writing. New York: Oxford University Press, 1988.

38 Auditory cortex: Disterhoft, J. F., & Stuart, D. K. 1976.Trial sequence of changed unit activity in auditory system of alert rat during conditioned response acquisition and extinction. Journal of Neurophysiology, 39 [2], pp. 266-281.

39 "Paw cortex": Kalkaska, J., & Pomeranz, B. 1979. Chronic paw denervation cause an age-dependent appearance of novel responses from forearm in "paw cortex" of kittens and adult cats. Journal of neurophysiology, 42, pp. 618-633.

40 Amputating a raccoon's fifth digit: Rasmussen, D. D. 1982. Reorganization of raccoon somatosensory cortex following removal of the fifth digit. Journal of Comparative Neurology, 10, pp. 313-326.

41 Somatosensory reorganization in the cortices of raccoons: Kelahan, M & Doetsch, G. S. 1984. Time-dependent changes in the functional organization of somatosensory cerebral cortex following digital amputation in adult raccoons. Somatosensory Research, 2, pp. 49-81.

42   Patrick Wall's prescient suggestion: Wall, P.D.1977. The presence of ineffective synapses and the circumstances which unmask them.

43   Philosophical Transactions of the Royal Society of London, Series B; Biological Sciences, 26 ,pp. 361-372.fifteen times as dense as those on, for instance, your shin: Heseltine, E., 2000. How your brain sees you. Discover, September, p. 104.

44   The poor brain was hoodwinked: Paul, R. L., Goodman, H., &Merzenich, M. 1972. Alterations in mechanoreceptor input to Bradman's areas I and 3 of the post-central hand area of Macacamulatta after nerve section and regeneration. Brain Research, 14, pp. 1-19.

45   Roughly eight to fourteen square millimeters: Merzenich, M. M., & Jenkins, W. M. 1993. Reorganization of cortical skin representations
   Of the hand following alterations of skin inputs induced by nerve

46   Injury, skin island transfers, and experience. Journal of Hand Therapy, 6. pp. 89-104.
   Neuroscience land Marc: Ibid.

47   Inputs from the radial and ulnar nerves: Merzenich, M. M., Kaas. H., Wall, J. T., et al. 1983. Progression of change following median nerve section in the cortical representation of the hand in areas 3band 1 in adult owl and squirrel monkey Neuroscience, 10, pp.639 -665.

48   "Complete topographic representation'': Merzenich & Jenkins, 1993, p. 92.

49   "Completely contrary to a view of sensory systems ": Merzenich, Kaas, & Wall, 1983, p.662.

50   "Hubel and Wiesel's work had shown just the opposite"; Hubel, D.H., Wiesel, T.N.1970. The 1970. The period   of susceptibility to the physiology, 206, pp. 419 – 436: Hubel, D. H., Wiesel, T.N., & Le Vay, S1977.

Plasticity of ocular dominance columns in monkey striate cortex. Philosophical Transactions of the Royal Society of London, Series B: Biological Sciences, 197 (29), pp. 377 -409.

51   The representation of the hand : surface representations

In areas 3b and 1 in adult owl and squirrel monkeys. Journal of Comparative Neurology, 258, pp. 281-296.

"Differences in lifelong use of the hand s''; Merzenich, Nelson, & Kaas, 1987, p. 281.

52   Amputated a single finger in owl monkey: Merzenich, M. M., Nelson, R. J., Stryker, M. P., ET a. 1984. Somatosensory cortical map changes following digit amputation in adult monkey. Journal of comparative Neurology, 224, pp.591-605.

53   A single, continuous, overlapping representation: Clark, S.A.,
Allard, T., Jenkins, W. M., & Merzenich, M. M. 1988. Receptive Fields in the body-surface map in adult cortex defined by temporally
Correlated inputs. Nature, 332, pp. 444-445;
Allard, T., Clark, S. A.,Jenkins, W. M., & Merzenich, M. M. 1991
Reorganization of Somatosensory area 3b representations in adult owl monkeys after Digital syndactyly. Journal of Neurophysiology, 66, pp. 1048-1058.

54   When the fused digits were separated: Maligner, A., Grossman, J. A., Rebury, U., et al. 1993. Somatosensory cortical plasticity in adult humans revealed by magnetron paleography. Proceeding of the National Academy of Sciences of

the United States of America, 90,
pp. 3593- 3537.

55   Adult visual cortex seemed just as
capable of reorganizing: Kaas, J.H.,
Krubitzer, L. A., Chino, Y.M., et al.
1990. Reorganization of
retinotopic cortical maps in adult
mammals after lesions of the retina.
Science, 248, pp. 229-231.

56   Experiment on four of the Silver
Spring monkeys: Pons, Garreaghty,
Et al., 1991.

57   "New direction of research";
Ramachandran, V. S., & Blakeslee,
S.
1998. Phantoms in the brain: Probing the
mysteries of the human mind New York:
William Morrow; Ramachandran, V. S.,
& Rogers-

58   Ramachandran, D., 2000. Phantom
limbs and neural plasticity.
Archives of Neurology, 57, pp. 317-320.

59   The term phantom limb: Herman, J.
1998. Phantom limb: From Medical
knowledge to folk wisdom and back.
Annals of Internal Medicine, 128,
pp. 76-78.

60   Fee the missing appendage:
Ramachandran & Blakeslee, 1998;
Ramachandran, V. S., Stewart, M., &
Rogers-Ramachandran, D.1992.
Perceptual correlates of massive cortical
reorganization. Neuroreport, 3, pp. 583-
586; Ramachandran, V.S. 1993.

Behavioral and magnetoencephaloographic correlates of plasticity in the adult human brain. Proceedings of the National Academy of Science of the United States of America, 90, pp. 10413-10420.

61 Invaded by nerves from the genitals: Robertson, I. H. 1999. Mind Sculpture: Unlocking your brain's untapped potential London: Bantam Press, p. 54. For excellent reviews of the clinical aspects of plasticity, see: Robertson & Murre, 1999, and Robertson, I. H., 1999.

62 Setting goals for cognitive rehabilitation. Current Opinion and Neurology, 12, pp. 703-708.

63 Double by 2050: Taub, E., Uswatte, G., & Pidikiti, R. 1999.

64 Constraint-induced movement therapy: a new family of techniques with broad application to physical rehabilitation—a clinical review. Journal of Rehabilitation Research and Development. 36. Pp.237-251.

65 Speed and strength of movement: Ibid.

66 "Neurological injury, including stroke": Taub, E., Miller, N. E., Novak, T.A., et al. 1993. Technique to improve chronic motor deficit

67 After stoke. Archives of Physical Medicine and Rehabilitation, 74, pp. 347-354.

68 In just two weeks: Robertson, I. H.,
    & Murre, J. M. J.
    1999.Rehabilitation of brain
    damage: Brain plasticity and
    principles of guided

69 Recovery. Psychological Bulletin,
    125, pp. 544-575.

70 Improvement on standard tests of
    motor ability: Kunkel, A., Kopp, B.,
    Muller, G., et al. 1999. Constraint-
    induced movement therapy

71 For motor recovery in chronic stroke
    patients. Archives of Physical
    Medicine and Rehabilitation, 80, pp.
    624-628.

72 Patients who had lost the leg: Taube,
    Uswatte, & Pidikiti, 1999.

73 Brain changes in six chronic stroke
    patients: Liepert, J., Miltner, W. H.,
    Bauder, H., et al. 1998. Motor
    cortex plasticity during Constraint-
    induced movement therapy in stroke
    [patients. Neuroscience Letters, 250,
    pp. 5-8.

74 Changes in the brain's electrical
    activity: Kopp, B., Kunkel, A.,
    Muhlnickel, W., et al. 1999.
    Plasticity in the motor system
    related to

75 Therapy-induced improvement of
    movement after stroke. Neuroses-
    Port, 10, pp. 807-810.

76 "Induced expansion": Taube,
    Uswatte & Pidikiti, 1999.

77 Left aphasic: Pulvermuller, F., Neininger, B., et al. 2001. Constraint-Induced therapy of chronic aphasia after stroke. Stroke, 32 [7], pp. 1621-1626.

78 Largely destroyed their Wernicke's area: Weiller, C., Sense, C., Rijntjes, M., et al. 1995. Recovery from Wernicke's aphasia: A

79 Positron emission tomographic study. Annals of Neurology, 37, pp.723-732. Accompanied by cortical reorganization: Liepert, J., Bauder, H.,

80 Wolfgang, H. R., et al. 2000. Treatment-induced cortical reorganization after stroke in humans. Stroke, 6, pp. 1210-1216.

81 Reported a similar finding: Buckner, R.L., Corbett, M., Schatz, J., Et al. 1996. Preserved speech abilities and compensation following

82 Prefrontal damage. Proceedings of the National Academy of Sciences of the United States of America, 93, pp. 1249-1253. Tactile discrimination tasks activate the visual cortex: Sadato, N.,

83 Pascal-Leone, A., Graf man, J., et al. 1996. Activation of the primary visual cortex by Braille reading in blind subjects. Nature, 380, pp. 526-528.

84 Superior tactile sense of the
    congenitally blind : Cohen, L. G.,
    Celnik
P., Pascal- Leone, A., et al. 1997.
Functional relevance of cross modal
plasticity in blind humans. Nature, 389,
pp. 180-183.; Musso,
85 M., Weiller, C., Kiebel, S., et al.
    1999. Training-induced brain
    plasticity in aphasia. Brain, 122, pp.
    1781-1790.
86 For the good of millions of stroke
    patients: Taub, E., & Morris, D. M.
2001. Constraint-induced movement
therapy to enhance recovery after
stroke. Current Atherosclerosis Reports,
3, pp. 279-286.